Healthy Me

Healthy Me

Discovering Personal Health & Healing Naturally

YVONNE LONGMATEY

MBA, BSN, BS, RN, CHC

ParahBooks

Printed in the United States of America

Library of Congress Control Number: 2019931239

ISBN 978-1-7335660-0-1

Published by ParahBooks
a division of Parah Wellness
710 Dacula Road, Ste. 4A, #121
Dacula, GA 30019

www. ParahWellness.com

For everyone in pursuit of
personal health & wellness, this
book is for you!

CONTENTS

PREFACE

Welcome to a new "Healthy Me"!

We all desire optimal health and wellness. The path to this can be different for everyone, but can be traveled with determination. I share valuable lessons from my personal experience with you in this book. These concepts will help you travel faster in your own journey of discovering personal health and healing.

In recent years, there has been an upward trend in the occurrence of many debilitating diseases. The range can be anything from diabetes or hypertension, to the various forms of cancer. Quality of life is key. You don't only have to pay attention when a situation is of a terminal nature. Not being able to take a few brisk steps without stopping to catch your breath can get in the way of enjoying a good quality of life. Inability to moderately enjoy a treat without the intervention of a shot of insulin to manage outcomes can be challenging. It's very easy to get complacent with managing the symptoms of a disease, to an extent of finding it unnecessary to make lifestyle changes that can enhance quality of life. On the journey we're about to embark on together in this book, we'll take a look at some building blocks and foundational principles that will give us an added wellness advantage.

Many factors have been shown from extensive research studies to be possible causes of certain diseases on the rise today. Some of these factors have also been shown to potentially worsen existing conditions. It's important to acquire knowledge about everyday helpful strategies you can incorporate into your lifestyle that will naturally promote great health for you. In an era where information can become overwhelming, many people are stunned by the large amounts available, some of which have raised safety concerns over time. Typically, when it comes to the use of information, some people go overboard while others do the opposite, not realizing benefits from personal application. There is a strong need for understanding useful concepts illustrated in this book, that will help in analyzing certain key information. These great concepts will come in handy when you need to make choices on-the-go that can positively impact your health. Reading this book will help you to personally improve your health.

You are unique and have your own personal needs and preferences. In the end, the ability to make decisions that best fit you is essential to keeping you motivated and consistent in following through with the decisions you make. Generally, understanding what goes on around you is helpful when making your own beneficial choices. Whether this is related to shopping or travel, this general rule applies. When it comes to the body and health, it's no exception. The body is complex in nature, and its function is powered by several complex organ systems. Understanding details of how these organ systems work involves an extensive study with a focus on each of them. I can tell you from much studying, that as complex as the body is, application of certain basic concepts can help to enhance its performance.

In this book, I will focus on practical immune health-boosting strategies. I have found that if you focus on your immune health, you can and will improve your overall health. Boosting your immune health is important because when your immune system is in good condition, your entire body is stronger within and well-positioned to stay in top shape as well. Using my own experiences, I discuss personally derived concepts that will help you develop your own techniques and preferences for skillfully boosting your health. I discuss these useful concepts in ways you can relate to, and will be able to easily apply to your own specific situation. This approach to acquiring information has been proven to enhance long-term success, especially in the management of everyday choices that positively impact health. Additionally, I'll share many tips that will help you to practically obtain your own successes in improving your health without a need to invest excessive resources whether in time or money, in your pursuit of great health. Whatever your resources allow, you can make choices that will help you to enjoy better health.

INTRODUCTION

Your health is your most valued asset.
Be intentional in investing in it!

After going through a personal challenge in my own health where it seemed impossible for doctors to find diagnoses for what was going on in my body, I had to go on a journey that would ultimately lead me to come up with "tools" that would help my situation. I began to apply these concepts in various ways which helped boost my own health in the tough situation I found myself in. I grasped the fact that my personal, educational, and professional experiences were necessary and needful in this journey, and I am thankful that the dots from all these areas of my life connected well in leading to the development and application of these concepts which I share throughout the book. This book is about concepts I believe are essential to health and healing. I discuss my personal experience of health and healing as I elaborate on these concepts.

We tend to hear a lot about the things we need to avoid to stay in good health. However, not as much emphasis is placed on what we can do to empower our bodies to stay in good health. With a backdrop from my personal journey, this book will take you on an expert but very simple approach that will challenge you to visualize the role of your immune health from a different angle than you currently see it. You'll gain an understanding of my useful health-boosting concepts explained in creative ways that would challenge you to pursue better health in practical ways. Additionally, I will touch on some of the very simple tools and resources you can use around you. Soon, you'll be able to apply these concepts daily and arm your immune health with enhanced strength and ability to defend you. You can improve your health and wellness without breaking the bank!

In my many years of practice as a Registered Nurse and Biologist, my knowledge of the disease process, its natural progression, and expected end results, have been mind-boggling in comparison to what I have seen many times in practice. This is especially true because I have witnessed certain instances where expectations based solely on knowledge in comparison to actual outcomes have posed many variations. These have left room for many other possible reasons and thoughts. Typically, many disease processes begin with a germ (pathogen) entering the body as in the case of certain infections. However, there are also many other diseases that are triggered by the body's exposure to an accumulation of factors that are needed for the disease process to start in an individual who can be easily affected by these factors. Let's call whatever could start the disease process, whether a germ or an accumulation of factors, a "trigger". This individual who is vulnerable to, or can potentially be affected by the "trigger" would be known as the susceptible person. For this discussion, let's simply classify the "triggers" as "intruders" of the body's normal state.

When this "intruder" makes its way into the human body, the susceptible individual who is more likely to succumb to the disease is typically a person who also has several other factors or conditions within their body that weaken their ability to respond effectively to this "intrusion". These weakening factors favor the multiplication of the "intruder" to an extent or level where it can cause harm in its new environment. In the example of the intruder as a "germ", once it reproduces itself and creates a condition in this individual's body, that would favor the disease's progression, it takes over. Then, the disease is produced in the individual. One major factor that can easily promote the "germ" in the direction of causing its corresponding disease is a weak immune system. The body's immune system is made up of the body's various "tactics and equipment" that help it to protect itself from "intruders", as in the case of the "germ" mentioned.

There are some people who are exposed to a "germ", that do not develop a disease because of their very strong immune system, which is able to ward off any potential effects from this "germ". Sometimes these people with strong immune health may even come down with the disease initially, but the period of the disease for them is short, as compared to others with a weak immune system. This is because their bodies are typically able to quickly marshal defenses that ward off effects started by the "intruders" within their bodies. Is it possible for you to be among this group of people with strong immune health? The answer is, yes, if you can empower your immune system to effectively perform its function.

Furthermore, boosting your immune health is important because there are many diseases today whose absolute cause or cure have not been found despite extensive research effort. In certain instances, specific factors have been cited as possible causes of some of these diseases, from studies of disease processes, which continue to evolve. I have personally witnessed patients who were expected to die from certain diseases within a specific duration live longer and healthier beyond the given time periods estimated by their doctors. I have also seen patients admitted to the hospital with seemingly minor diagnoses, turning quickly down paths that have led to their deaths. I have pondered over this for many years, and I see that although we do not always have control over the external exposures that trigger certain disease processes, we can take steps to decrease our chances of being affected by some diseases. A major way of doing this is to strengthen your body's immune health via your everyday lifestyle choices and routines. You can effectively do this when you understand how your choices holistically affect your body. Your health is your most valued asset. Be intentional in investing in it! No one is promised another day, but we have the option of paying attention to things that can improve the state of our health. This is important because success in all aspects of life heavily depend on our health. Give your best to taking care of your health, and all other areas of your life will obtain benefits from this action!

Acquisition of knowledge is invaluable to taking good care of ourselves. I have witnessed many frequent repeated hospitalizations that I believe could sometimes have been easily prevented with knowledge of what could have been done in certain instances. Many times, these have been heartbreaking, more so when related to the lack of knowledge about basic prevention techniques, availability of resources, or the lack of motivation to do some of the simple but potentially helpful things.

Through knowledge, you can provide your immune health with a further boost. This boost can give your body an enhanced ability to defend you from potential health "intruders". Surely, you can take steps that count toward better health! From this book, you'll be able to take on a new approach to optimal health that focuses on what you can do to empower your immune health, so you can stay in shape and be productive in other aspects of your life. Not only will you realize an understanding that will help you put elaborated concepts to use in your own wellness journey, but you'll also gain an empowering ability to take advantage of some of the very simple and inexpensive resources around you, even from your own kitchen, to achieve this purpose. I believe everyone can do this, and reading this book will take you a step in the right direction of boosting your health via your daily routines.

CHAPTER ONE

The Body Can Heal Itself (My Personal Journey)

The body can heal itself if provided the right conditions that trigger the process of healing.

On a Sunday morning in May 2012 around 7 a.m., everything changed for me. I woke up that morning, had what I call my "quiet time", as was my usual routine, and walked downstairs to get breakfast ready for myself and my family. We were preparing to attend church service which was to start at 10 a.m. that morning. As soon as I took a gallon of milk out of the refrigerator, I passed out in the kitchen, as I'd later come to find out.

I opened my eyes to see my husband kneeling beside me in the kitchen, asking if I was okay. I assured him I was okay, while trying to make sense of why I was laying on the floor and why he was asking me if I was okay. He could not make sense out of it either, but later told me he knew there was something terribly wrong when he saw me laying on the floor. He said he heard a loud, strange, sound from upstairs, like something falling. He ran downstairs, only to find me laying on the kitchen floor. He said he was very grateful to God that I did not show any outer signs of bruising when he found me, although he was sure everything was not alright.

My husband followed his instincts and immediately got me into the car. We headed for the Emergency Room (ER). At the ER, a wide range of tests were performed on me. These included an extensive blood work and a CT scan of my head. They all came back negative, except for an elevation in my white blood cell count. From my personal understanding of the disease process as a Biologist and a Registered Nurse, I immediately anticipated my body was trying to fight something, although tests could not pinpoint to what exactly. I was sent home, with a recommendation to follow up with my primary physician. Tests did not reveal anything that needed my immediate admission to the hospital for continuous monitoring.

I went home with my husband, and little did I know that was going to be the beginning of a long 3-month battle for my health. Over the next 6 weeks, I began to run fevers intermittently during the day and at night. I felt very weak to where I could only lay in bed. I had to cancel all scheduled activities for my kids as well as my regular work commitments, to handle the feeling of constant weakness and to be able to take care of myself. I went to see my primary physician as recommended by the ER doctor. She also went on to perform extensive tests but could not find anything warranting immediate attention. All this while, my feeling of weakness was getting worse by the day. My primary physician then went on to refer me to specialists, including an Infectious Disease Specialist who conducted many tests as well. All these tests came back with normal results, indicating the absence of a problem in the areas tested. Amazingly, by this time, even my white blood cell counts were showing close to normal levels. My condition remained a mystery both to myself and the physicians who were taking care of me.

My situation posed a great challenge to me and my loved ones. The feeling of weakness was so overwhelming for me at the time that I could not physically do anything meaningful for myself, let alone for my family. I simply laid in bed and tried to comprehend what I was going through. I can tell you that after thinking deeply and knowing very well reasonable tests had been conducted by the medical team I had seen, I was left with only one option, and that was to call on whom I have known to be the greatest physician of all time, Jesus! I had a personal relationship with Him at the time, but it went even deeper, as I found Him to be the only one who could help me. I watched my husband and children do their best to take care of me; a picture of a role reversal in my opinion. I prayed specifically to God for Him to help me to make sense of this and to give me the strength to get back to my normal routines.

As a health professional, I had tons of thoughts of possible diagnoses running through my head based on the symptoms I felt, although the tests were indicating otherwise. However, I also felt strongly within my heart, not to put voice or words to the thoughts that were running constantly and aggressively through my head. I refrained from verbally assigning diagnoses to myself. Being a firm believer in Jesus and His word, I believe God's guidance afforded me the prompting not to do so. I personally believe my faith in Jesus Christ led my family and I, as well as a wonderful company of loved ones who prayed for me constantly to walk in hope, throughout this journey.

At this time, I began to pay attention to and apply the knowledge I had acquired personally, educationally, and professionally to test. I came up with concepts that would help boost my health. I realized I had come to a hard place where I desperately needed answers to what was going on in my body. As I started to walk along this road in order to rediscover health and healing over the next three months and beyond, I began to have an even deeper understanding of my body. I strongly believe that the in-depth knowledge I discovered during this 3-month journey and beyond, is totally attributable to the help of my friend, Jesus, who worked to help me understand and come up with many concepts I believe helped immensely boost and restore me to health. I believe my friend helped me to connect the many dots from my educational, professional, and personal experiences in a simple fashion. I share some of these concepts in this book and hope it will help you, or even a loved one, attain these great benefits as well.

One of the major concepts I discovered is the fact that God created the body in such a way that sometimes it's able to heal itself, just as it's able to start a disease process by itself. We may never be able to totally understand this phenomenon in spite of all we continue to learn about disease processes. But the truth is, it happens sometimes, and probably even more frequently than we realize. The key factor in this phenomenon is creating an "at-mosphere", or condition, that will allow the body to initiate and go through its healing process. These conditions can include nutritional, mental, emotional, and spiritual. Additionally, these multiple conditions interconnect and depend on each other. Many times, we separate them and tend to believe they have no connectedness to each other. This approach tends to cost us dearly, to the detriment of many people's health. In the same manner these conditions can join up to start the disease process, they can also interrelate to make the reverse happen. There can be an interconnection to provide the body with an environment that boosts its health.

As a Registered Nurse and Biologist, and especially when I take care of patients, I have always loved to think about the disease process, body systems, and how they relate to each other in functionality. I do this to better understand the needs of my patients and provide care that would afford them the best paths to optimal health and healing through whatever they may be experiencing. During this 3-month period in my own personal journey, the rubber met the road for me, as I got deeper in my own thought processes and tried to understand all that I had learned personally, educationally, and professionally. Keep in mind, that although I felt symptoms of a very sick person, I felt like nothing could be done for me because there were no pointers from medical tests as to what was going on within me. In the process, I personally experienced this concept which I simply summarize as: just like the body can start the disease process when conditions stir that up, it can also heal itself if provided the right conditions that trigger the process of healing.

Think about this, sometimes medications can provide favorable chemical conditions for the body to fight diseases. However, there may be times when it seems impossible to determine what the body is trying to "fight", or simply just finding the right medications to help it "fight", as in my personal experience. Under such conditions, it's needful to exhaust all other possible means to help the body, without giving up. There are even times when all the right medications are in place, but the body finds it hard to respond to these medications for a variety of possible reasons, which I believe could include emotional and/or psychological factors.

God is real. I have come to this conclusion based on my extensive acquisition of knowledge and experiences that are even beyond the scope of this book. These have led me to know and believe God is real. As we draw closer to Him and ask Him questions about mysteries that baffle us including those related to our health, He will guide us to find knowledge and give us clues, many times even beyond our acquisition of knowledge, so we can live and make wise choices and decisions that can lead us to living fulfilled lives that bring Him glory.

Through this personal journey, I came to an understanding and development of an approach to health and healing, which I personally term together, as "Immune-Strengthening Concepts". As a Biologist, the interest I have of how the cells, tissues, and organs in our bodies function is great. These are ideas I tend to visualize regularly. In these concepts, I use very simple scenarios to try to communicate a broad overview of what could sometimes be taking place in our bodies based on the kind of "conditions" we create by the little things we do daily. I focus on the importance of building a healthy immune system while going about our everyday activities in a smart, efficient, and seamless way. I explain how some of our daily choices can positively enhance and empower our immune health, in contrast to the other way around. These concepts are very much simplified to convey a wealth of helpful understanding.

CHAPTER TWO

Arm Your Body Right

The body does not work in a "vacuum".
It works with what we feed it to produce
the outcomes we see.

In my professional life, I can think of some of the many patients who have been told by a doctor that they only had so long to live. Some of these patients have defied odds and lived beyond the estimated periods. There is never an absolute explanation as to why this happens. On the other hand, I can also think of the sudden incidents of illnesses, and even sometimes death, in otherwise very healthy individuals whose great health have been proven from the standards of laboratory tests. Furthermore, I have come across people with many odds against them genetically, but who have made lifestyle choices that have afforded them paths to great health and happiness. Science is invaluable to health! However, it has limitations like anything else. As much as we've tried and continue to try, science has not been able to extensively explain everything, as there are stories that challenge textbook explanations. By gleaning from the experiences of others, in addition to acquiring various forms of scientific and non-scientific knowledge, we can help ourselves to make beneficial decisions. We can improve our health by the value of the choices we make.

Personally, I call our immune system "the body's defense hub". This is because of the role it plays in keeping us protected from disease. Generally, for a disease to occur in an individual, the body must primarily be exposed to an "intruder" that is foreign to it, as mentioned in the introductory chapter. This "intruder" must be armed with an ability to trigger or cause this disease, for example, a bacteria or germ. This "intruder" can also be an accumulation of factors in the body, enough to start a disease process. For example, let's say harmful substance levels from tobacco in certain disease processes, can progress to cause certain forms of cancer. Recall the fact that for an "intruder" to cause an actual disease in the body, environmental conditions within the body must be favorable for the disease process to start and thrive. The "susceptible" individual to this disease is the person with favorable conditions within their body that allows the disease process to start and thrive.

When the immune system is well-armed to carry out its defense function, it can create conditions within the body that do not favor the "intruder's" ability to successfully carry out the full process of the disease's development. Generally, a healthy, well-functioning immune system plays a major role within the body. A healthy immune system will create an environment that positions the body to be strongly defensive of "intruders". This environment tends not to favor progression of disease processes. In certain instances, even when it's started, a healthy immune system can prevent disease from advancing and continuing to the point of causing extensive destruction to the body.

There may be certain disease processes that do not conform to this norm. However, there are lots of disease processes that thrive in the body because of the body's failure to defend itself via a healthy immune system. This armed ability to fight "intruders" via its protective mechanisms, is the reason I call the body's immune system our "defense hub".

It's important to strengthen your immune system by providing it with what it needs to play its role in keeping you healthy. Think of your immune system as your system of defenses that help to prevent "intruders" from taking over your "home". Similar to a simple fence in your backyard, or your home monitoring system. When they are up and properly functioning, you feel safe and protected. However, when those "defenses" are broken and their capacity to function properly decreases, they can potentially pose as an easy attraction to intruders. This can be very dangerous to your home.

From extensive study and education, I have come to realize that there are many diseases, and many ways by which many of these diseases can initiate and thrive within the body. These get even more elaborate when it gets to certain specific diseases, most especially those whose specific causes cannot seem to be exhaustively explored. An extensive discussion of many of these different ways certain diseases could possibly be caused within the body would take us outside of the scope of this book. However, I need you to keep in mind the fact that these different possibilities exist. Additionally, the many different possibilities are a connection to the fact that humans may never be able to totally understand the cause of all diseases and how they progress, despite all the great and helpful things we do constantly to advance knowledge. There are paths of the unknown that still exist in this territory, and which is why an approach that could potentially take care of some of the unknowns, is needful in today's world. Adequately arming this "defense hub" can potentially help us, most especially in some of the unknown paths of disease initiation and progression, as I realized in my personal journey.

Every individual is a product of an intricate relation between their genetic factors and their environmental influences. The role genetics play is key, and it's a component we do not have control over. Genetic factors are deeply embedded within our makeup, and they comprise factors that have been passed down to us from our ancestry. However, environmental factors also play a huge role in influencing our lives, including certain diseases, how they start and advance within the body. In fact, genetics can influence the creation of certain conditions within the body that may also favor or hinder the initiation or progression of certain diseases. The truth, there are certain factors you may not have control over, but there are still other factors you can influence because of the choices you make. When you think about environmental factors within the context of this discussion and in a broad sense, think about the factors you choose to expose your body to on a daily basis. These can include food, activities, and the many everyday lifestyle choices you make.

The body does not work in a "vacuum". It works with what we feed it to produce the outcomes we see. Thus, goes the saying, "junk in, junk out". It's no wonder some people have very high energy when they eat certain foods and tend to get sluggish or slowdown in performance when they eat certain other foods. Our "defense hub" is an integral part of the body. Like the various systems in our body, it serves an essential function. Its function can be enhanced or weakened, based on the nourishment and attention we give to it. Our choices of certain environmental factors can enhance or diminish the ability of our "defense hub" in carrying out its essential role within the body.

In the creation of environmental factors that fuel and advance diseases within the body, this can be so subtle that it can very easily be overlooked. Additionally, because of the complex interactions of many environmental factors with genetics, it can get challenging pointing out any one factor as a sole "perpetrator", when it comes to identifying the cause of certain diseases. Let me use a backdrop of my own experience to elaborate on this. About 11 months prior to the start of the condition I found myself in, I had started school for my master's degree in an area of specialization that was completely new to me; business school. I had to put in extra effort to stay on top and be at my best. At the time, I was so focused on getting everything on my schedule perfectly taken care of, while pursuing my desire of getting all A's in graduate business school. Unfortunately for me, my educational background had solidly been from a science background and the area of business was new to me. However, I left no room to take it easy on myself during this stage of my life while learning new things. To further complicate this, my family had also just relocated to a new home. Sure enough, settling my family in our new home was a major task I underestimated while making the decision to start graduate school, working, and keeping up with other demands on my time. Not to mention the fact that there were other social commitments I had made, and I was also determined to keep up with every one of them.

A little about me in perspective, I have always been a high achiever. This tends to reflect in all areas of my life, especially when I pursue personal goals. I try to give my best in all things to ensure my very best outcomes. To me, this season of my life was not going to be different. I was determined to juggle everything excellently, alongside my new pursuit of educational advancement. I was not prepared to let anything suffer in the process, only to realize later I had a limit to this expectation.

As a nurse, this attitude translates into a personal drive of always striving to give my patients the best and treating them as I would want to be treated. It's an attitude that tends to bring me joy, and a personal sense of fulfillment. I bring this attitude into everything I put my hands to, and taking care of my family is no exception. Unfortunately, I struggled to stay at the level of perfection I desired. This brought on a new level of constant stress as I worked effortlessly in all roles to continue to stay exceptional.

I would later understand I was almost always in a constant state of anxiety in my effort to be extremely successful in all these areas of my life. As is the case with most of us, I was too busy to even find time to notice I was stressed, let alone find time to deal effectively with the high levels of stress. I simply didn't pay attention to myself. I continued this pace until my body could no longer keep up. Later, I reflected on this and I realized as a believer that the enemy had taken advantage of this situation, and had fueled the high levels of stress in my life. I had not learned to rest in Jesus and trust Him completely to help me through. Yes, I prayed for His help, but I thought I had to do it all by myself, and I did not realize that truly resting in Him would also mean simply doing my best and leaving outcomes to Him. Furthermore, I was so busy that paying attention to my nutritional intake was not a priority, even though I knew very well that it was necessary to position my body in a good place so it could adequately handle stress. It is one thing having the knowledge you need, and a completely different thing purposefully using the knowledge to your advantage. The latter should always be our goal, or else we could leave too much room for unwanted but often possibly preventable outcomes.

In my situation, a complex system of environmental factors was at play in making my body susceptible to "intruders", and for that matter, perpetuating the disease process. This is because the resulting high levels of stress from my choices only served to further weaken my "defense hub", in addition to the neglect of its proper nourishment.

I look back and see that I could have done a much better job. It was necessary for me to take good care of my body so it could in turn, keep up with the demands necessary for my sustenance. There are many of us who have very busy lifestyles, and often these lifestyles are demanding on our bodies. I can confidently tell you that if you give yourself some "breaks" to take care of your body, you'll be thankful you did. These nourishing breaks will fuel your body to go with you for a longer haul than it would if you neglect it. Paying attention to the body's "defense hub" is important. Allowing prolonged stress can and will do more harm to you than good. The body's "defense hub" can be strengthened or weakened by the environmental factors we expose it to, depending on the choices we make.

There are lots of research studies that support the fact that most diseases that are reported to physicians each day are stress related. Many people experiencing mental stress tend to realize a huge negative effect of this on their overall health if not properly and promptly dealt with. This is because of the negative effect stress can have on the body's "defense hub", compromising its ability to adequately function in its role of fighting "intruders". In fact, a research finding attributed as much as 60% to 90% of visits to the physician as having stress-related causes.[1] I could go on and on with stress and its associations with disease. In fact, from heart disease to gum (periodontal) disease, stress can play a major role. Stress can weaken the immune system greatly, leaving the body with an environment that favors the course of diseases from start to thrive, when the body is exposed or faced with an "intruder".

There are many factors that contribute to stress. Oftentimes, these factors are overlooked. Worry can be a major fuel to stress. It only complicates conditions both externally and internally for us, although it does not change whatever we may be worrying about. It is no wonder the Word of God tells us that we should not worry and that it only causes harm.[2] This harm is usually much more than we can completely point our fingers to immediately at the time of worry. The great thing about the body is that an exposure to "intruders", even chemicals[3], will not always lead to a disease.

Building a strong "defense hub" is essential for good health. Paying attention to environmental factors that can enhance the health of our immune system is helpful to purposefully providing the necessary boost, needful for this key system in our body to continually carry out its functions effectively. In subsequent chapters, you'll find out some of the various ways by which you can purposefully arm your "defense hub" to function more effectively.

CHAPTER THREE

A Scavenger Hunt Within: Aim For This!

*You only benefit from the actions you take.
Don't overlook the seemingly simple things
in life and pay dearly for the neglect later.*

Often important but very easy to overlook, one of the major ways of boosting the health of our immune system can be paying close attention to fighting free radicals that are formed within our bodies. Free radicals are highly charged molecules, that can easily react with other molecules such as those normal molecules within the body, and cause damage to them. These free radicals can accumulate within the body in many ways. One significant way of accumulation is internal, from inside of the body in the form of byproducts from the functioning of bodily cells. Another means is from external sources as from air pollutants, what we eat sometimes, and much more.

In a functional sense, these free radicals are atoms or a bunch of atoms that have unpaired electrons, causing them to be unstable. For illustrative purposes within this context, picture atoms as the littlest basic particles. These particles can be from simply anything that makes its way into our body, or already existing within the body. Free radicals in their basest forms have this attribute of atoms as well. Generally, these atoms have even smaller components called electrons, which love to live in pairs. When the electrons of an atom live in pairs, they are happy, stable and content. Unfortunately, free radicals have electrons that are unpaired. These unpaired electron components make them "angry", with a desire to snatch electrons from other surrounding atoms. Because of this, they tend to be very reactive, always in search of other electrons so they can be totally paired. I call them very lonely atoms seeking friends aggressively.

Their high need and capability to react and pair those lonely electrons they have, make them very dangerous. In fact, these atoms can easily set up a cascade when they "snatch" electrons from stable atoms around them, leaving these other atoms in an unstable state like they previously were. In this "snatching" process, they attain stability while causing their opponent to become unstable and in turn repeating the process. Keep in mind the fact that the atoms they are snatching from can be components of vital cells, tissues, or organs of the body. When this process occurs continually within the body from an accumulation of free radicals not taken care of, it can lead to damage to otherwise healthy cells. This results in a possibility of allowing diseases easier access to the body as these healthy cells are damaged by the action of free radicals.

Atoms typically combine with others to form a group of atoms known as molecules. Any atom or molecule can get into a reactive state with unpaired electrons, even oxygen, which we need and use for many functional processes within our bodies.

Oxygen in an unstable state, with unpaired electrons, can also easily stimulate and initiate the formation of free radicals because of its highly reactive nature, when it interacts with some molecules within the body. This cascade of reactions can be very detrimental to the body's health when they occur in some of the most vital components such as the DNA. In this way, free radicals can sometimes serve as fuel in the development of certain diseases. There are many diseases, such as certain cancers, certain heart conditions, and many others, whose initiation and progression could be benefiting from cellular malfunction or cellular death which is stimulated by the action of free radicals. As attention is given to the possible role of free radicals in the disease process, research work will continue to unearth some specifics.

There are also chemically reactive groups of molecules that contain oxygen as a component of their free radical components, such as superoxide and peroxide. These are generally known as the Reactive Oxygen Species. When present in this state, the oxygen can serve to speed up the action of free radicals. With this idea of oxygen as a "catapult" to the action of free radicals, some light can be shed on why free radicals are also produced during exercise, a time when the body uses lots of oxygen to produce energy.

Keep in mind that exercising is a highly beneficial activity to the body and its function. During exercise, the body uses large amounts of oxygen to increase metabolism. In the process, there are various by-products inclusive of free radicals, as the oxygen helps in cellular functions such as the burning of body fat in certain instances, to produce more energy. In this process, some of these resulting free radicals include the Reactive Oxygen Species due to the high amounts of oxygen at play in the process of exercising. The body has a way of ridding itself of these exercise-produced free radicals, most especially in healthy well-nourished individuals with healthy "defense hubs". Hence, that form of free radical production does not typically pose a concern in such individuals. As in exercising, there are many normal and needful everyday activities we're involved in, that also feed into the process of production and accumulation of free radicals within the body through no fault of ours. For this reason, it's very important that we take care of also increasing the body's ability to rid itself of free radicals from within itself so we can reduce their potentially harmful effects. When it comes to free radicals, it's not just a matter of whether or not they are produced, because they will always be produced to some extent. Rather, our focus should be on how well they are taken care of so they do not pose great danger within the body over time.

The presence of excessive amounts of free radicals in the body can lead to a condition known as oxidative stress. Oxidative stress can occur in the body when the levels of free radicals produced within the body are at a much higher rate than the body is able to cope with. The body finds itself struggling to offset the potentially harmful effects caused by their presence within the body. I introduce the *concept of balance*, as pertaining to strengthening our immune health. Balance is essential in many processes, both internally and externally, and can promote good health. That is the reason why maintaining a balanced lifestyle, inclusive of what we eat, is necessary for maintaining good health. Scientifically, oxidative stress has been said to be one of the major causes of disease development in the body[1,2], as well as "accelerated" aging.

The body can counteract oxidative stress by neutralizing the effects of these free radicals with antioxidants, as from what we consume from foods rich in them. This is a key reason why eating foods rich in antioxidants is a major way to prevent oxidative stress from sustaining itself within the body. These antioxidant-rich foods can work to "scavenge" potentially toxic free radicals, thus disarming them of their harmful effects and detoxifying the body. Doing this can help the body to decrease the rate at which it ages, as well as prevent certain diseases from starting and thriving within the body. It's needful to give attention to eating foods rich in antioxidant properties so we can reap the essential benefit of scavenging free radicals from their action.

There are many ways by which the body can generate and/or accumulate free radicals within. Of great significance is the fact that some of these free radicals are easily generated from everyday activities, even certain activities very useful to the body. An example is that from exercising as mentioned earlier. Sources of free radical accumulation within the body can include harmful environmental toxins such as smoke, radiation from the sun and other sources, etc. These toxins can be both naturally occurring as well as from man-made chemical pollutants. The body in a "sick" state can also produce free radicals at high levels. In other words, every individual would have certain levels of free radicals in their body no matter their activities or lifestyle, however careful they may be. I say this because it is impossible to isolate ourselves from everyday activities such as driving, where we sometimes inhale some levels of smoke from cars all around us. Even walking across a "polluted" environment can potentially expose us to a certain level of free radical accumulation from inhalation, not to mention exposure to harmful radiation from the sun, which is also a great source of Vitamin D.

Let me mention that when at all possible, it's best to plan for the times you go out to enjoy the sun, to coincide with times when harmful rays are radiating at a minimum. This is generally before 10 am or after 4 pm on an average day. However, I also know that many times, our schedules do not permit strict planning for minimal exposure. Because of this, we experience some levels of exposure to harmful radiations. Furthermore, the necessary benefits we obtain from physical exercise is invaluable to our health. Exercise helps to circulate oxygen to vital organs of the body, increasing its overall strength and performance. Hence, this reflects in our feeling of a boost of energy, strength, mood, and overall vitality when we exercise regularly. The body also needs nutrients from food to produce energy for function, as well as nourish itself to maintain performance at optimal levels.

Most of us do our best in minimizing exposure to pesticides while shopping for foods. We try to pick the best foods from the grocery store by choosing items with minimal possibility of pesticide contamination and chemical processing, and so much more. However, no matter how hard we try, there are still days when we must eat in restaurants where we do not have all the possible control checks from the farm to our plates. I could go on and on. Exercising all the possible precautions is very good and important and should be done. I'm only saying that it's near impossible to do just every right thing. Many times, we end up with some levels of free radicals within the body. Hence, the necessity of focusing on empowering our body to "scavenge" some of these free radicals is needful to boosting our immune health. The amazing news is that God has armed the body with the capability of taking care of these free radicals if we provide it with the right conditions, such as the right nutrients or right actions in this context.

Boosting our intake of foods rich in antioxidants are a great way of empowering our bodies with the ability to "scavenge" these free radicals. Remember how "unstable" and "lonely" free radicals are? How they are seeking stability by "snatching" electrons from stable atoms? This is where antioxidants become friendly to these free radicals by providing them with the electrons they need for stability. Unlike most other atoms in the paths of these free radicals when they make their way into the body, antioxidants possess an amazing feature. Antioxidants are stable whether they have unpaired electrons or not. Hence, they can act "friendly" by donating electrons to these free radicals which in turn become stable, without becoming unstable themselves to carry on a cascade of relative reactions. These antioxidants thus neutralize the dangerous actions and/or reactions of the free radicals within the body, thus preventing cellular damage that can occur because of the action of these free radicals.

We know from earlier discussions that it is almost impossible not to have free radicals in the body, as they can be produced either from necessary, beneficial, activities we carry out daily for our very sustenance, or from "pollutants" we can encounter because of our everyday activities. Yet still, others choose to introduce free radicals into their bodies because of the gratification they derive from certain activities, related to making these free radicals abundant in their bodies, as in smoking. In addition to the possibility of causing certain diseases such as those mentioned previously, aging is a very common side effect of the activities of free radicals. This is another major reason for which working on "scavenging" them from within the body can help to boost not only good health within but the evidence of it without. A beautiful glowing skin can be achieved by simply paying attention to this simple action. Think about the impact of smoking on the skin of people who smoke. This is the result of the action of large amounts of free radicals inhaled via smoking.

On its own, the body can produce some antioxidants as in the production of glutathione, a powerful antioxidant.[3] As reflected in its name, this powerful antioxidant consists of three major amino acids, namely, glutamine, glycine, and cysteine. The body naturally produces and regenerates glutathione within it. Like other antioxidants, glutathione can help the body to rid itself of free radicals. Good thing, it's naturally produced within the body. From its basic component list, a well-nourished healthy individual would be in a better position to better arm the body with nutrients it would need to produce such valuable antioxidant. Thus, placing the body in a better position to scavenge some of its free radicals. Everyone can help boost this production of antioxidants within the body by providing the right "environment" via what we eat or the actions we take. There are many enzyme systems within our bodies that can scavenge these free radicals if we simply boost their production.

Of equally great importance is a number of antioxidants we can provide our bodies with via our diet. For this chapter, I limit discussion to a few major ones, Vitamins C, E, and beta-carotene (the precursor to Vitamin A). These antioxidants are richly available in most of our fruits and vegetables. As the old saying goes, eating a rainbow (variety of colors) of fruits and vegetables help to make sure you are covered. This saying is true, even in boosting our immune health. There are also many foods that are rich in other sources of antioxidants.

Vitamin C is a water-soluble vitamin, richly available in most of the fruits and vegetables we eat. Green leafy vegetables such as spinach and kale, broccoli, colored bell peppers, etc., as well as most fruits such as kiwis, strawberries, citrus fruits like oranges, etc. are a rich source of Vitamin C.

The National Institute of Health (NIH) states that Vitamin C has been elevated as a means of helping and/or treating many health conditions because of its role as an antioxidant and the role it plays in immune function.[4] The NIH provides information and basic facts on nutrition and supplements such as Recommended Dietary Allowance (RDA) for Vitamin C intake. For Vitamin C, this averages about 60mg for adult non-smokers. However, smokers have a higher requirement of about 35mg more than that of non-smokers.

The National Cancer Institute highlights studies that have shown some successes when cancer patients have been treated with high doses of Vitamin C, with some even done intravenously.[5] They have carefully mentioned drawbacks of these studies in certain instances when Intravenous Vitamin C treatments were given alongside with chemotherapy drugs and side effects were realized. Most healthcare workers who give IV infusion would attest to the fact that this is not uncommon, as there are many drugs that work very well within the body as individuals, but do not go well together when administered in IV form, with other drugs due to incompatibility issues. Thus, these studies are not surprising, most especially given that there is so much positive result obtained from their studies when the Vitamin C in IV forms have been administered alone, leading to some studies to conclude that high-dose IV Vitamin C in patients with cancer have shown an improvement in their quality of life and physical state as well as other cancer-related symptoms.[6] This further supports the fact that Vitamin C is an immune health booster, as typically, the immune system of cancer patients tends to be compromised, the reason for many of the symptoms that are exhibited, and their susceptibility to infections and other diseases.

Note though, that the U. S. Food and Drug Administration has not approved the use of IV high-dose Vitamin C in treating cancer or any other medical condition.[7] More research is needed in this area, so certain hidden potential benefits can be unearthed. Also, be aware when utilizing research information, that conclusions would usually be conservative, as research is always carried out with certain limitations given consideration. Hence, although there may possibly be lots of research studies supporting a concept, researchers would usually refrain from making absolute conclusions. Furthermore, for any research study, there may be other research works that support otherwise, typically fewer in numbers and with limitations as well. It is thus very important to analyze research holistically, stringing many and others that relate, to come up with personal conclusions when utilizing research-based information.

It is no wonder that the U.S. Food and Drug Administration tends to be cautious in making any conclusions, as in the use of IV Vitamin C in treating cancer patients, although positive results have been noted in some research work. Of great importance is the fact that health research work is invaluable to our health. It helps to further support what we usually know is beneficial to our health, or even give us certain pointers or clues to explore the unknown with potential benefits.

Orally consuming Vitamin C from your diet can serve to make this potent immune health booster available in your bloodstream and allow you to obtain its wonderful health benefits. When unable to consume enough from foods, some people take Vitamin C as a food supplement. Consuming foods rich in Vitamin C can make a significant contribution to boosting your immune health, given such substantial significance of it. Making that purposeful extra daily effort may be well worth your time. Consider making fresh fruits and vegetables an important and necessary part of the produce in your kitchen. Remember that even if you take Vitamin C as a food supplement, the body absorbs nutrients best from food, and the extra fiber you obtain from these are invaluable to your health in aiding digestion and the overall health of your digestive system. So, in addition to your supplement if you take that, eat fresh fruits and vegetables. Remember the general rule of eating at least 5 servings of fruits and vegetables daily. Not only can you get Vitamin C from your fruits and vegetable, but beta-carotene, another major antioxidant. This can also be obtained from green leafy vegetables as well as many other fruits and vegetables such as carrots, squash, peaches, cantaloupe, yams, etc. Think of brightly colored orange fruits and vegetables as in the color of carrots and peaches, to connect beta-carotene and where it can be obtained. It's important to know that Vitamin A is formed from beta-carotene, although Vitamin A has no antioxidant properties by itself. The key is beta-carotene, so make your diet count.

Vitamin E, another powerful antioxidant, can also be obtained richly from most edible fruits and nuts, whole grains, fish oils, fortified cereals, and again, fruits and vegetables such as avocados, olives, apricots, and our green leafy vegetables. It helps to protect cells from the oxidative stress produced by free radicals and works well in combination with Vitamin C to provide greater antioxidant properties. Do you see lots of skin protectants, certain sunscreens and lotions fortified with Vitamin E? This is because of the protective effect it offers the skin from the sun's UV rays and other harsh environmental conditions.

Now let's take this a step further, the popular phrase "beauty comes from within". We can take better care of our skin by consuming foods rich in Vitamin E and other antioxidants. Growing up, I remember the hypothetical link of carrots to good eyesight and skin. The Vitamin A that forms from beta-carotene helps with great eyesight. The beta-carotene also provides an antioxidant action that leaves our skin beautiful. Therefore, in addition to enjoying the benefits of Vitamin E in our skin care products, let us consume enough of it, together with beta-carotene, to make our outward beauty stem from within and be long sustained.

By now you may have noticed a pattern. Green leafy vegetables span across all major antioxidants mentioned. As a general personal rule, the darker and more brightly colored the fruit or vegetable, the higher the probability that it would be richly loaded with antioxidants. The greens are always valuable when thinking about the various arrays of colors. Think about these tips when in the grocery store aisles and load your carts with various colors of fruits and vegetables.

As a personal help, I love to take an "inventory" of my diet weekly and make plans to incorporate some of these antioxidant-rich foods in my daily menu. I do my best to include green leafy vegetables, avocados, brightly colored fruits and vegetables such as carrots, peaches, broccoli, whole grains, beets, and the many others, in my diet. The more, the better. I always say that I thank God that there is such a wide variety that even if you do not like certain fruits and vegetables, you can try to find others you may like. There are so many great recipes out there you can take advantage of and enjoy some of these amazing fruits and vegetables. Keep in mind when adopting new recipes, that it's necessary to be sparse on condiments, or find healthy alternate substitutes, or even avoid some, as well as decrease salt and sugar to tolerable levels whenever these are excessive. Of course, occasionally, I go the whole length, but try to maintain a level of control … as we all do.

As simple as this sounds, eating foods rich in antioxidants will go a long way to boost your immune health. Let your kitchen be the source that is richly loaded with these to help you achieve the well-needed boost of your immune health in its role of scavenging antioxidants. You only benefit from the actions you take. Don't overlook the seemingly simple things in life and pay dearly for the neglect later. Do what it takes, and start to plan something meaningful from today onwards.

CHAPTER FOUR

Put Out The Little Fires

No one fights for a prolonged period
without getting tired. The body is no exception.

O ver the years through my educational and professional journeys, I have discovered that some of the information that stay with me the longest and tend to be
most useful, consist of those I'm able to make mental illustrative
connections to. For this reason, I'd love to use this approach in
fostering an in-depth and lifelong understanding of wellness
concepts that will stick with you and help you in making daily
decisions that would boost your health. Understanding is key!

When I think of the inflammatory process within the body,
I find the concept of small fires in a large campground a great
way of describing the process. Think of the body as the large
campground. The body systems and/or organs can be compared
to a lot of different groups of people or individuals lighting fires
at this campground. Keep in mind that these little fires may be
initially necessary, maybe to keep warm, roast a marshmallow,

etc. However, if these fires aren't attended to, they can "blow up" and get out of hand. If not contained well, these fires that get out of hand will cause injury or even death to these campers who had been obtaining benefits from them initially.

Now, that is what the inflammatory process compares to within our bodies. The initial little fires are a good thing. However, if not well controlled and contained by the campers, it can get out of hand and pose a great danger to the same people who initially obtained great benefits from it. Likewise, the body naturally uses the inflammatory process to "protect" itself by getting rid of what it perceives as "foreign" to it. Keep in mind that this "foreign" agent is also known to us as an "intruder" to the body. Generally, the body regards this "intruder" as an "attacker" and tries to respond by safeguarding its environment. Initially, the inflammation process is very helpful to the body, as it sets "little fires" in various parts within the body as needed to defend itself, or simply to keep it in good shape. The body mounts these "little fires" as defenses, whenever it feels or senses an "attack" in any part of its members (could be within tissues, organs, etc.). This sensed "attack" could come from outside of the body such as a viral or bacterial invasion (pathogens), or even irritants such as smoke, harmful chemical irritants from the air, etc. The sensed "attack" could also be from within the body, as in dead or damaged cells from an injury or anything that potentially causes death or harm to cells, and which could many times be anything that is not normally present within the body's environment.

This phase of the inflammation process is what I call an "innocent start". During this phase, the body's major goal is to protect itself. The phase can occur for various reasons. For example, at the start of an injury to get rid of dead cells. It can also occur as a means of defending itself from an outside invasion. The body needs this phase. It's a healthy phase and a natural mechanism by which the body protects itself. It's also generally known as the acute phase of the inflammation process.

What I term as "little fires" comprise of the whole cascade of biological events the body stimulates at a site of the perceived attack, to fight and maintain its otherwise "normal state" that had existed before the arrival of what it perceived as an "intruder". An example of this can typically be seen in the initial phase of let's say an injury. Think of the warmth and redness that quickly starts up when you have a cut on your hand. This is great, and it's the body defending itself to keep its normal state as prior to the cells getting injured from the cut.

Acute inflammation is usually short-lived and resolves rapidly by itself because of negative feedback mechanisms that are stirred into action in the process. The body gets rid of the "intruder" and heals itself in the process. Now, as in the case of the "little fires" at the camp, this is normal, and it is really what we want. We need a strong ability of the body to defend itself.

However, when this initial inflammation process is not well regulated or well contained by the body and extends itself beyond the initial phase and becomes prolonged, it moves into the chronic phase of inflammation, which is a stage that is detrimental to the body. This chronic stage of inflammation can typically get the body into a diseased state or even worsen an already existing condition. Now, also imagine autoimmune diseases, such as rheumatoid arthritis and many others, where the body starts an immune response against its own healthy tissues because it begins to get "confused" and perceives its own healthy tissues as "intruders". With such diseases, the body begins to "self-destruct" as the inflammation response is kicked off, and typically progresses from the acute phase into the chronic phase, as the body stays "confused", seeing its own healthy tissues as "attackers". This results in the chronic disease state, which we typically see in many of these autoimmune diseases. The resulting type of autoimmune disease also depends on which part of the body this phenomenon occurs, and the effect produced by the "self-destruction" process.

There are many instances where inflammation begins in the body, but the body safely resolves the process by itself, many times in the acute phase. Often times, we're not even aware of it happening while the body is resolving it. In many of these instances, it is because the body has been provided with a conducive environment that affords it the necessities to turn off those "little fires" (inflammation, especially at the initial phase). This prevents the "little fires" from self-sustenance and progression into a chronic phase to cause a disease.

Studies have shown that chronic inflammation has even been associated with the development of cancer. In the disease process of cancer development, substances active in the inflammatory process, known as inflammatory cytokines, have been associated with tumor formation.[1] These inflammatory cytokines are molecular substances that signal and assist in mobilizing cells in an immune response action, as in initiating an inflammatory response at an injured bodily site, or where a perceived "intruder" is sensed. Thus, to find cytokines in the process of tumor formation, this would be an indication of the body's attempt at fighting off a perceived "intruder". An ability to successfully complete this mission would be a plus in overpowering this "intruder".

There are many common chronic diseases that have been associated with some aspects of the inflammation process, as in cardiovascular (heart) disease, diabetes, autoimmune diseases, to mention a few. Even depression has an activity of inflammatory cytokines, busily playing a role in its progression. In the case of cardiovascular diseases, risk factors such as high blood pressure, smoking, high levels of bad cholesterol, can significantly contribute to a buildup (atherosclerosis) in the inner walls of blood vessels of the heart, and which the body perceives as foreign to it ("intruder"). Through the inflammation process (putting out "little fires"), the body begins to form its own "wall" or "capsule", to keep this buildup away from its normal blood flowing through its vessels. By this action, the body tries to protect itself from its perceived "intruder". Over the course of time, the formation of these "walls" or "capsules" cause a narrowing of affected blood vessels with such consequences as heart attacks in certain individuals. In some instances, these "encapsulated" buildups would break off and their contents would interact with certain components of the bloodstream, leading to blood clot formation. Blood clots which make their way into some vessels and parts of the body can be dangerous to health. These can cause serious incidents, as in some cases of stroke.

There is extensive ongoing research as relating to statins, a cholesterol-lowering drug that seems to decrease arterial inflammation, according to the American Heart Association (AHA).[2] Other drugs are being investigated, to see if they can reduce arterial inflammation, and decrease the risk of heart attack and stroke.

Strengthening your immune health, which is a key player and influencer in the body's inflammatory processes, can be an important means of enhancing your overall health. A major area in research as pertaining to heart disease seems to be towing along the lines of finding a means of curbing inflammation in the arteries. There are ongoing attempts to find drugs that work best to prevent some of these heart-related diseases.

Many studies have shown links between obesity and lots of chronic diseases, including Type 2 Diabetes. Of significance is the fact that intertwined with these is the inflammatory response, also active in situations of obesity. As a matter of fact, inflammatory signaling pathways have been found to be associated with processes involving insulin resistance.[3,4] Thus, we see inflammation "represented" in pretty much so many chronic disease pathways.

Inflammation plays a major role in the aging process, for which reason it is so important to boost immune health as one grows older, to better arm the body to age gracefully, while also decreasing chronic disease occurrences. Unlike healthy acute inflammation, chronic inflammation keeps the body in a prolonged "fighting state" as the inflammation process is perpetuated.

No one fights for a prolonged period without getting tired. The body is no exception. After a long period of being in a state of chronic inflammation, it gets worn out, and the strength of its immune health declines. People with certain chronic conditions tend to have weakened immunity and become susceptible to infections and other diseases. For example, a person admitted to the hospital for long periods to treat a chronic condition could easily end up with another condition if certain preventative measures are not put in place. This can happen because the individual's decreased immunity becomes an "open door", attractive to other diseases over time, and some of which could even be hospital-acquired.

The great news is, even chronic inflammation can resolve over time if the body is armed with the right environment. As a matter of fact, there are lots of "intruders" that our bodies ward off seamlessly without us noticing because we do not feel any pain or receive any obvious signal of something having gone wrong. Making good choices one moment at a time, whether it's in what we eat, or the activities we choose to carry out by the minute via our daily routines, we can make a difference in providing the right environment within our bodies, in helping it to be effective at handling inflammation.

When armed with an ability to stay in good condition, the body can handle inflammation well lots of the times. For this reason, it's vital for us to consume the right nutrients and take on routines that help to keep the body in top health.

Research supports the fact that even tumor cells adapt very well, and thrive in an environment that has poor nutrients, and insufficient oxygen. [5] From my own experiences and the incidents of people I have coached, I can confidently tell you that the little choices you make every day can afford you the necessary tools to arm your body well, and naturally. These little choices can help your body to become proficient at initiating acute inflammation and effectively putting out those "little fires" when it needs to defend itself. Easy to overlook, effective everyday choices can decrease your body's chances of staying in perpetual chronic inflammatory states.

Even if you have a chronic disease, it's possible to assist your body to decrease its chances of staying perpetually ill by taking advantage of the little opportunities that come your way, to impact your health positively via your daily choices and routines. In addition to increasing your intake of foods rich in antioxidants, boosting your intake of foods that are rich in anti-inflammatories are very helpful. These two tend to work hand in hand.

While antioxidants and anti-inflammatories can work hand in hand, some helpful possibilities of benefiting from both worlds can be from the consumption of some basic spices, rich in anti-inflammatories, antioxidants, or both. As a simple example, the sulfur-containing compounds in garlic has great anti-inflammatory properties. We tend to think a lot about our fruits and vegetables, which is very important, but what is of additional importance, is our spice rack. Many times, the spice rack is not visited as much, but kept as décor in most of our kitchens.

Very often, we tend to hear about foods that should be consumed in minimal quantities such as processed sugars and deep-fried foods, just to name a few. Worth noting, these foods have great potential to fuel the chronic inflammation process, with many being contributory factors to leading chronic diseases such as heart disease, and many others. For example, high levels of bad cholesterol (LDL) from deep-fried foods soaked with high levels of saturated fats make cholesterol abound in the bloodstream. This excessive amount of bad cholesterol in the bloodstream has a high potential of sticking to blood vessels as in the plaque formation example, with potentially harmful consequences, as in the cause of certain strokes. A high consumption of deep-fried foods has been linked to a corresponding high occurrence of type 2 diabetes and heart disease (more elaboration in Chapters 10 & 24).

Of course, it's great, and certainly alright to give yourself those occasional sweet treats and some deep-fried foods. Keeping these occasional is key. When the body is consistently armed with great nutrients most of the time, occasional unhealthy treats do not have what it takes to overwhelm and overpower it into a low state of self-defense as pertaining to immune health within this context. You can make choices that position you with immense confidence to give yourself an occasional treat without feeling guilty. Chapter 11 will help you to do just that, and on your own terms too.

Picture an ability to boost your body's health with so many nutrient-rich foods to such an extent that your occasional "dilution" with "junk" foods would not even make a significant impact on the overall state of health of your body. Now, that's what I believe you should consider desiring and working your way up to.

Carefully consider increasing your intake of foods with high anti-inflammatory benefits, to empower and enhance your immune health. There are many research studies that have shown people benefiting from consuming foods rich in anti-inflammatories, and yes, even some people in managing certain chronic conditions. Unless you are allergic to them or are taking medications that contraindicate you consuming them, carefully consider trying some foods rich in anti-inflammatory properties. It would be worth your time.

Additionally, God is amazing and has created a wide variety of them. Surely, you'll find one that works for you if only you are willing to try and stay open to exploring the numerous options out there. As a tip, on a regular everyday dietary intake, when in doubt, look out for colorful vegetables and fruits, and don't forget the amazing greens. You will not be disappointed.

CHAPTER FIVE

What Fuels Those Fires?

Be mindful of your "Breaking Point" and that of those around you. This will lead to healthier expectations, key to building and enjoying healthier relationships.

L et me mention briefly here, that it's very important to pay attention to the nutrients in the food you eat. This is because you can use this attentiveness to your advantage when it comes to handling the inflammatory processes in your body. You can even help to decrease the potency of certain "fuels" of the chronic inflammatory process by this action. If taken seriously, your health will greatly benefit from this action. There are many factors that enhance chronic inflammation in the body. I focus on a major one whose impact can be very detrimental to health but is often underestimated. This is chronic stress. I also discuss practical and effective ways of dealing with this potential health hazard. Note that for this analogy to help provide a better understanding, I use oxygen in a negative sense of fuel, in comparing to the dangers of chronic stress to our health.

We know that what fuels any fire is essential to the fire's long-term sustenance. Oxygen plays a major role when it comes to starting and sustaining fires. Even in our kitchens, we see how easily the fire from our gas stove would go off by just turning off a little knob that disconnects the source of fuel which would otherwise keep the fire burning for as long as we would need it sustained for cooking. Oxygen boosts and provides fuel for the fire to burn continuously, in addition to igniting the fire. Firefighters use a variety of tactics to curtail fires during fire outbreaks. One of the major ways by which they try to contain the fire in an outbreak is by cutting off the oxygen source of the fire so it can be more easily contained.

In the method of cutting the oxygen source, the use of a dry chemical extinguisher contained in tanks is common. These dry chemical extinguishers are typically in the form of a foam. Other times, they are comprised of some dry chemical powders and nitrogen gas, utilized as a means of activating the chemicals into action during emergencies.[1] The chemicals typically work by "suffocating" the fire to death. This is achieved by layering the foam or powder over the fire and disconnecting the fire from the oxygen in its immediate environment. When this technique is effectively carried out with the objective of "cutting" the fire off from its source of oxygen, the fire goes out. This is what we typically see as the result. In this analogy, we see that the effectiveness of the technique in cutting the fire off from its source of oxygen is critical to success in putting out the fire.

With this analogy in mind, a major fuel to the chronic inflammation process, and what we usually would also see reflected in chronic disease progression, is stress. It is very easy for us to overlook the harmful effects of chronic stress and let it linger for lengthy periods in our bodies. Stress tends to "creep" easily into many people's lives. Due to its subtle nature, stress can find its seat in the body as an "unwanted guest" by staying without being noticed for as long as it's permitted. Over a lengthy period, it takes over a "room" in the body, in the form of chronic stress. It would typically stay until it's purposefully evicted. For this discussion, I'll label chronic stress as the "creepy unwanted guest" so you'd be able to visualize really what it is. Chronic stress can cause so much harm. It's important to make sure you do not allow it to find a seat, let alone, a room in your body. The creepy nature of chronic stress arms it with an ability to cause damage without being noticed, making it very dangerous.

How many people do you know, including yourself, who may be stressed but would deny its existence right away, when asked? Very few people acknowledge stress when asked if they are stressed. From my experiences, I realize a major way of finding out if you are allowing stress to creep into your life, is to take occasional pauses to reflect on your own life. Check to see if there are any new routines you have introduced, and which you have not yet gotten used to. Are these causing some concerns for you? Once you become aware of that, it is necessary to put measures in place to handle those concerns, and remember, once that is done, you do not have control over the outcomes. Ensure your best in doing your part, and let that worry out the window of your house. This is not the easiest to do, and it calls for a frequent reexamination of yourself, particularly your thought patterns, and dealing with concerning issues. De-stressing is discussed more thoroughly in Chapter 6.

You may be wondering what could be termed as stress, and that's very important. To simply help you visualize an analogy, think about trying to break pieces of twigs from different plants. The twigs would be plucked from various positions of these plants. There would be some level of pressure you'd apply to each twig that it's able to handle, preventing it from breaking off from its parent plant. However, there would also be some level of pressure for each twig, beyond which it would not be able to handle, allowing breakage from its parent plant.

You'd realize that much older twigs, usually picked from the lower part of a plant, tend to withstand higher pressures and take relatively more intense pressures to break, as compared to younger, fresher, twigs, closer to the top of these plants, which tend to break more easily with relatively lesser pressure. Again, you'd realize that carrying out this same experiment on an oak tree would be much different than a small rose plant. Furthermore, the fragility of the twigs would be different in different seasons of their life cycles. The present season can affect the twig's ability to withstand applied pressure. For example, whether it is winter or summer, can make a difference with regards to how fragile a twig would be on its plant. Of equal importance is the fact that a well-nourished twig may withstand higher pressure before it breaks, compared to another twig of the same size that is malnourished.

Now, equate these twigs to different people, and the other factors to the various situations and conditions that make these people different, or influence their overall situations at different times or stages in their lives. Stress, in its simplest form, can be explained as whatever may be overburdening to an individual. However, we realize that the level at which this could cause an individual to "break" would be different for different people. This is because each person perceives stress differently and has different "breaking" points. These limits beyond which one would "break" can also be complicated by the various demands already existing in the lives of different people. Additionally, some people can handle more "pressures" than others. Typically, in a healthy individual, this capacity to handle "pressures" tends to increase over time when it's effectively dealt with as it comes in. You need to take appropriate measures to put plans in place to effectively stress.

Most importantly, each one of us is different, and have different abilities to handle different situations. It's important to always put that in perspective when relating to others, whether at home, work, or in any other relationship. Reciprocally, this will also help us to be more understanding of others and make us more willing to tolerate other people who may not be wired to handle as much as we have grown accustomed to handling at any given time or season of our lives. We would be able to build better relationships with this understanding, by not having unreasonable expectations whether of ourselves or others. Be mindful of your "Breaking Point" and that of those around you. This will lead to healthier expectations, key to building and enjoying healthier relationships.

Note that although emotional, stress causes responses within the body that can immensely affect it negatively. There is some occasional level of stress that is necessary for effective "performance". This type of stress gives us the required "push" to complete tasks, as in meeting deadlines. This kind of stress is very healthy in keeping the body engaged in its functions. Now, when stress becomes long lasting as in the one that keeps you worrying and staying awake at night, it tends to be the "breaker of the twig". This is what I am describing as a major cause of chronic stress. Beware of this kind of stress. At this stage of stress for most people, they would most likely have moved into a phase of needing to deal with chronic stress. Some common manifestation of chronic stress can be in headaches, muscle tension, acne, peptic ulcer disease, or a compromised immune system.[2]

A compromised immune system is a major gateway to simply an endless list of possible diseases, as it provides a fertile environment, where chronic inflammation can thrive and perpetuate itself. Of equal significance is the reality that such environments can very well feed into any potential health complication, worsening an already struggling state of health in the process. These factors can work together to affect the health of an individual. It's very important to pay attention to taking care of these "little fires". Earlier, I mentioned an important example of taking on responsibilities that will not go beyond your breaking point. Additionally, always find opportunities to work on increasing your capacity to handle more, as you take on responsibilities that are tolerable for you at any given level or season. This will allow you some time to make room to accommodate growth that will not break you.

In recent statistical studies, it has been shown that about 43% of all adults suffer health-related issues that are stress-related, and in fact, a good 75-90% of all visits to the doctor are for conditions that are stress-related.[3] To further show the relative importance of stress to the state of our health, it is worth mentioning that stress has been linked to six principal causes of death (lung disease, accidents, cancer, heart disease, suicide, and liver cirrhosis). Stress has been declared a workplace hazard by the Occupational Safety and Health Administration.[4]

We need to be attentive always, and deal with getting rid of this "creepy unwanted guest". It calls for frequent evaluations of our lives for chronic stress. For each one of us, depending on the relative demands in our lives, the frequency for re-evaluations may differ. For some people, a daily reevaluation is necessary to put in some measures that will help prevent chronic stress. Sometimes all it takes is putting in coping mechanisms to deal with work overload or better scheduling for family activities to fit into other demands. Remember, stress usually creeps in silently, and many times stays as long as it wants to without being noticed, while causing lots of havoc in many lives. Go the extra mile, get to know the signs, and have a plan in place to deal with stress. This can make a great difference in enhancing your immune health.

Remember one reason stress is easily overlooked is the fact that it is typically emotional, psychological, or mental, whichever makes it easy for you to visualize. It is not one that is easy to physically detect. It has the capacity to stay for a long time in the "mental domain", as I'll state for this discussion, and thrive successfully. However, the body's functional systems are interconnected and typically intricately interdependent on each other. Whatever goes on in your mind does somewhat affect your brain, which in turn can stimulate actions in the nervous system. Bear in mind that one major way the brain and the nervous system communicate and carry out their functions within the body is by stimulating the action of chemical and electrical "messengers" that can travel to different parts of the body to trigger desired activities.

Do you remember the phrase "laughter is the best medicine"? This isn't just true on a social level, but also on a biological level as pertaining to the physiology of your body. This is because laughter can mentally put the mind at ease, and stimulate the body to release hormones called endorphins, which have a pain-killing effect. This is only a little example to demonstrate the importance of a stress-free, healthy state of mind. Simply put, stress weakens the immune system.

When you think of stress, think also about the hormone cortisol. Cortisol is a steroidal hormone, which together with epinephrine, another hormone, are major regulators in what we call the fight-or-flight response. Chronic stress puts the mind in a state of constant anxiety and can stimulate the body into a state that mimics carrying out the fight-or-flight response perpetually. The purpose of the fight-or-flight response is to allow the body to carry out a series of system-wide functions that prepare the entire body to take care of itself in a case of "emergency". For example, running away from a wolf trying to attack you. These series of functions result in making energy readily available to parts of the body that would be involved in carrying out a response, whether it's your legs running at top speed, or your hand taking a large stick at close range to hit the wolf. When the body prepares to carry out this fight-or-flight response, a boost of energy availability is necessary to help complete the mission at hand. Blood sugar (glucose) is a major source from which the body generates the energy needed to carry out such responses.

For this reason, a system of actions is initiated which makes glucose readily available in the bloodstream. This is where cortisol plays a major role. One of the major functions of cortisol is helping to make blood sugar available in the blood, while at the same time decreasing stored glucose in the muscles, to accommodate the extra glucose needed to be released into the bloodstream. Do you see how this could affect the demand for insulin and its need in diabetics? With an abundance of glucose in the bloodstream, do you also see how stress could possibly trigger type 2 diabetes in an individual whose body may be overwhelmed with the need to effectively regulate sugar in their bloodstream? In recent times, along with the prevalence of other major chronic diseases, stress has become a major contributor to a rise in type 2 diabetes.

Our body's functions are interdependent, and it's the reason we need to pay attention to some of these "little fires". While this goes on, epinephrine contributes to blood vessels narrowing while blood is channeled to the organs preparing to carry out the response, causing the heart to beat faster as it works harder to pump blood into circulation.

In the wolf attack example, your body can respond in various ways. You may choose to fight this wolf, or simply escape by running away. Your body will then calm down and all the activities that occurred during the period of anxiety will resolve after you've completed your chosen action. Except while on a hunting adventure, anyone who sees a wolf suddenly will be unsure of what to do initially. So much anxiety and fear will set in, which will then stir up the body's fight-or-flight response. Your body calms down and "recoups" once it has successfully completed an action that stems from its fight-or-flight response. Generally, in a healthy individual, the body is wired to handle these occasional occurrences and stay in shape. Thus, the short-lasting periods of stress, as in what will drive us to complete that project, study for that test, prepare for that meeting, etc., are great, and actually boost our immune system and health, as it helps to keep our brains active and "things in motion".

Our bodies are wired to deal effectively with these short periods of stress. However, in a healthy individual, the body begins to run into problems when this mode is sustained for a long period of time, moving into a chronic state of stress. In this state, the body has no time to calm down, and it's in a constant state of "preparation for fight-or-flight". Also, in this state, cortisol is abundantly produced. Not only is it in turn making blood sugars high in the bloodstream, but it tires out the organs that are producing it (the adrenal gland in the endocrine system). This, in turn, affects many other organs that are trying to keep up with the cycle, thus, "wearing" the body out.

Another great significance in all these as pertaining to the health of the immune system relates to the mechanism of action of the hormone cortisol. Cortisol is a key player in regulating inflammation in the body. Think about times when you buy over the counter steroidal creams for your skin. You may have also experienced a doctor prescribe such creams for you or someone you know when there is a skin disease that has direct relation to inflammation with which resolving the inflammation could result in some relief. I use the example of the skin because it's easy to visualize and relate to. Many of these over the counter anti-itch skin creams that target inflammation contain some low levels of cortisol (or hydrocortisone). Whether it's someone you've seen with allergies or acne, you may have come across the use of cortisol in some form. This makes it easy to relate steroids to inflammation. Applying this a step further, cortisol also plays a key role internally, in regulating the inflammatory process within the body. A research study has pointed out the fact that cortisol, when not allowed to properly serve this function, could lead to inflammation getting out of control.[5, 6]

Chronic stress has been shown to be a culprit in negatively impacting the effectiveness of cortisol in its ability to regulate the body's inflammatory response, as it lowers the tissue's sensitivity to this hormone.[7, 8] In this study, healthy adult participants who were exposed to the common cold virus showed differences in their likelihood and in the actuality of them developing the common cold. Participants who had been exposed to lengthy times of stressful events were the most likely and were those who yielded to the infection and illness. The researchers discovered from their findings that yielding to the cold infection was due to the participant's immune cells not being able to respond to hormonal signals that normally regulate inflammation because of their lengthy exposures to stressful situations.[9, 10] Those who were not able to effectively carry out the needed immune response ended up with the illness.

Remember the initial discussion of how the body carries out an immune response when exposed to an "intruder", in this study, the cold virus? This goes even further to support the fact that the body's ability to carry out the immune response successfully would be a high factor in determining whether or not an individual would experience a disease, when exposed to the germ that causes that disease. We find from this study and many others, support of the fact that exposure to chronic levels of stress decreases the strength of the immune system in effectively carrying out its protective function. We also see how high levels of cortisol is released into the body during chronic stressful periods. With a decrease in its effectiveness at this time, the body responds with an even greater production in its attempt to make up for the ineffectiveness. It's comparable to shouting louder to be heard when someone is trying to calm an already tensed situation involving people, with loud noise already present within the environment. Not very helpful, but hard to think of any other way at the time.

In the case of excessive cortisol production via various stimulating actions, it further fans into compromising the strength of the immune system in a process that was initially started as a good thing to help the body. This is typically the case in the body, starting with a well-meaning intent until it gets out of control. Hence, we see that chronic stress is very relevant, and needs to be dealt with so it doesn't serve as "fuel" to any potentially threatening condition in the body, whether it's an already existing condition or an unexpected exposure to an "intruder". There are many ways by which we can intentionally unwind and relax the body, to keep it from exposure to long periods of stressful situations, whether it's from work or home. It is very important that we pay attention to intrusions from chronic stress and take necessary steps daily, to "unwind" and stay calm no matter what.

CHAPTER SIX

Killing A Major Enemy:
My Personal Experience

Being healthy is not just a physical state but also relates to the health of your mental, emotional, and spiritual domains.

W e've seen so far, that chronic stress is a serious enemy to our health, and it should not be entertained at all within the body. The cause of chronic stress is very different in the lives of each one of us. It is thus very important for every individual to pay attention to the "buttons" in their personal lives that bring on chronic stress. My experience of what led to me passing out and being sent to the emergency room is one worth reviewing. This had happened at a very crucial time in my life when I was busily pursuing educational advancement amidst other demands. Sure enough, this was a game changer for me. I now look back and realize that obviously, one of the major fuels to what happened was allowing myself to nurture chronic stress, which opened the door to other problems that doctors could not even diagnose at the time.

Many times, chronic stress creates a mental condition where your mind seems to be in a constant state of anxiety. This eventually affects your ability to stay calm, as your spirit is also affected by much "noise" resulting from the anxiety. Likewise, in my case, this constant state of anxiety affected my spirit and my ability to keep calm. It also interfered with even my peaceful communication with my Maker, a very pertinent relationship I hold dearly. I believe wholeheartedly that God's divine intervention is the very reason I'm alive today. In Chapter 1, I described my personal situation of what got me into the Emergency Room, with doctors unable to diagnose what was going on with my health.

From my description of the circumstances that surrounded this occurrence, I can confidently tell you that I "overstretched" myself and did not have the proper tactics in place to help me better handle all the demands I had to deal with. I had put myself in a position where chronic stress had set in. Now I look back and realize that I should have learned to equip myself with strategies that would have prevented me from getting into a state of chronic stress. These strategies that I discuss have worked well for me and have been amazing. Putting these in practice, I was able to complete my degree with my desired academic goals, while concurrently handling other competing demands, and also keeping up with enjoying a better quality of life.

I won't even say that I am the best at using these strategies at all times, but I can say that I take them a day at a time and consciously do my best to use them. Sometimes, I miss using them promptly when needed, but I make the necessary effort to fall back on them. I can tell you from my own experience, that if you also choose to use them daily, you'll be amazed at how useful and handy they come in over time, with conscious continual use. This stride is an important step I have made, in battling chronic stress and enjoying a healthier life mentally, emotionally, spiritually, and physically.

Your physical health has great connection to your emotional and mental health, which also have great ties to your spiritual health. Being healthy is not just a physical state but also relates to the health of your mental, emotional, and spiritual domains. Dealing with chronic stress, its effects, and ways to efficiently manage it, requires taking great care of all the different domains of our lives because of how much they feed off of each other. This highly substantiates the importance of being totally healthy in every domain. Most significantly, remember, it's the daily steps you take to successfully manage any stressors in your life, that make the most impact in preventing chronic stress. Chronic stress can be the major "fuel" that potentially "ignites" and even sustains possible "fires" that affect your health.

Helpful Combat Strategies

These are tactics I have found very practical and highly useful to me in this area of my life, as pertaining to dealing with the prevention of chronic stress. They can be very useful to you as well if you consider taking just a little bit of effort to incorporate them into your lifestyle. The benefits are amazing and absolutely worth the try.

Prime Times

Every day, I find my prime times to be the start and end of my day. This is because these times really affect how the entire day, as well as the next, would be for me. Therefore, I find starting and ending my day right to be very important to me in carrying out my daily routines. This is a key personal focus, where strategizing right is helpful for me in preventing chronic stress. There are so many things that compete for our time from the moment we wake up to when we fall asleep.

Once the alarm clock goes off, we wake up and begin to rush to the first scheduled activity. Think about that, the "alarm" clock. An indication of noise, something alarming, needing our immediate attention, a disturbance, and we tend to follow our day just in the manner the alarm clock wakes us up. For me, finding a calming routine when I awaken, has been vital to taking good care of my mental, spiritual, and emotional states. This may be different for everyone. Some examples can include sitting and reading the Bible; exercising, whether outdoors or indoors; drinking tea out on your porch while watching birds; or simply any other quieting activity of your choice. You can come up with your favorite list and even vary them. Personally, no matter the choice I make from my list, I always include praying and reading my bible, as I have found this to be most helpful to me. Starting my day with a quieting routine has great benefit to my physical health and it will help yours as well.

Rushing to a busy schedule and running around in an anxious state the moment an alarm clock goes off, can predispose the body to chronic stress, which can be detrimental to the body's health. More so, when this mode becomes an accepted daily routine, the immune system can be weakened as chronic stress creeps in over time. Quieting the body at the start of the day helps to position your body and mind in a calm state, making it better able to handle any potential stressors the day may present it with.

Night and day have great interdependence and interconnection with each other. It is of equal importance to also talk about my nightly routine. How I end my day affects how well I rest at night, which also influences how I start my day. In the same vein, how I start my day has a great impact on how my day will go, which also impacts my mental and emotional state, and ultimately, my physical health. I realize that different people have different sleep needs in terms of hours needed to rest the body properly. Generally, sleeping well at night helps the body to calm down and relax. Some people can sleep for about 6 hours most weekday nights and are able to function effectively without being grumpy in the morning. On the other hand, I would not in any way try to be like the person with a 6-hour sleep need. I realize I do well with a good 7-8 hours of sleep at night and could use even more if I had the time. However, I know this works best for me, although there are some days when I am not able to get those hours of sleep due to pressing demands. Knowing my body performs better with 7-8 hours of sleep, I do well to plan for this need ahead of time, and discipline myself to make time for those hours of sleep. I try not to stay up late whenever possible. I generally factor in my 7-8hrs nightly sleep need when I plan for bedtime, when making daily plans. This helps me to start my day in a well-rested state of mind.

Like the average person who must juggle work, family, and other demands, I tend to have a packed schedule on weekdays. With all this in mind, starting my day well rested and right is essential for me to be able to function at maximum capacity. Remember that everyone has different sleep needs for their body, although the recommended for an adult at night is 8 hours. You can easily find yours by beginning to note how many hours of continuous sleep at night you had, on days when you have woken up feeling rested and showing a good overall ability in handling the demands of your day without feeling fatigued, most especially within the first few hours of your day. You can confirm this also, by consistently sleeping those hours and reevaluating your daytime performance. You'll find what works best for you. I realize that although I did this before the incidence of me being admitted to the ER with a seemingly impossible to diagnose condition, I did not fully put into perspective the importance of how this routine affected my overall health. Looking back then, and connecting to the incident, I now see this not only as a routine but a necessary part of my daily life, in ensuring that my body is well taken care of, to stay in good health.

Now, due to the personal importance I attach to finding a "calming" moment in spite of the busy nature of my daily routines, I plan and discipline myself to wake up early in the morning, a little before my routines start, to have what I call my "quiet time". It also makes sense for me to plan to sleep as early as possible whenever I can, so I'll be able to make room for my "quiet time". This time is very precious to me, as it helps me to get my mind in a relaxed state, even before the busy routines kick in. This "relaxed state of mind" is what many try to achieve using various relaxation techniques. Muscle relaxation techniques are particularly great to learn and use routinely. For example, an ability to take deep relaxing breathes in a tensed situation can be very helpful. I particularly love my morning routine, as I find it useful to my emotional, mental, spiritual, as well as physical domains. It takes care of all relevant domains in positioning me well to start my day.

I have found what works best for me, and I hope what I describe as my "quiet time", will be helpful to you in finding yours. You can consider giving mine a try. You'll get to enjoy the great benefits I obtain from it. During this time, I personally pray by closing my eyes and talking to God about my day. I also read scriptures from the bible and meditate on them as I pray, so my mind is equipped with words that empower me to start my day. One of my favorites is from Philippians 4:13[1], "I can do all things through Christ who strengthens me". I resort mentally to some of these verses during the day when I encounter challenges. I connect to them and declare them in difficult situations in the Name of Jesus! It's powerful, and it works wonders for me.

Through my "quiet time", I start my morning with a great way of connecting with my friend.[2] I realize this is also a great way of reassuring myself of the strength I have available to me to complete my day. Via this routine, I position myself with a mental, emotional and spiritual security that my friend is and will be with me always during the day. It gives me great confidence knowing that I have help to face any challenges I would encounter during my day. It helps me to take some guesswork off my table, that is usually accompanied by a consequent level of stress that comes with dealing with the unknown during the day.

At night before I go off to sleep, once I have completed my usual nightly routines, I also make time to mentally relax my mind, which I do again, just the same way I start my day. I have another "quiet time", much in the same way as I do in the morning. I do this right before I go to bed, generally dozing off to sleep thinking about a scripture I read. Again, this helps me to quiet down my spirit and emotions as I sleep, so I wake up not only physically rested, but mentally, spiritually, and emotionally rested and relaxed as well, properly positioned to start my day.

Starting and ending my day right is a thing I practice daily. I make every effort to do this, even if it means having to miss watching a TV show to make time to "quiet" down. It could also mean choosing to make enough time to meet my natural sleep hour needs for my body amidst competing activities. I try to do this because of the difference it makes in my overall health. I realize that doing this one day at a time helps me to not only experience the daily benefits I obtain emotionally, spiritually, and mentally, but I also realize the benefit of the positive impact this has on my physical health. Consider giving this a try.

Working The Plans Right

You might have thought about schedules, the moment you saw the word "plans". You're partially right in thinking along those lines. This has somewhat to do with some aspect of maintaining a schedule that works best for you. I have had many experiences coaching and helping people from all walks of life with varying goals and different limitations as pertaining to reaching these goals. For example, I understand very well that choices from a diabetic diet may be different in practice for a busy mom of four who works full time, in comparison to that of a busy dad whose job requires long hours driving a truck weekly across different states.

Each one of these people has unique circumstances surrounding their day, and which tend to influence their choices from foods available to them. However, we also realize that both individuals have something important in common, which is to ensure that they make choices with their meals that best help them in regulating their blood sugar on a daily basis. Both aspire to reach their goals, however, the practical steps they'd need to take in attaining these goals would be different for each of them, given that they have different available resources, whether in time, or the actual selection of foods they would have available at any given time, to make selections from. In other words, even if we have a common goal, we may have different resources available to us and would need to acquire strategies that position us to effectively manage these resources in attaining our personal goals.

Being effective with regards to putting into practice what they know, is important in making the difference as to whether each one of them would succeed in keeping their blood sugar levels within acceptable ranges for their condition or not. Being effective is key, and in the discussion of planning, I like to say that many people are skilled at planning but are not always able to plan effectively. Effective planning is key to everyday success, and in turn, decreases stress. This is because the more effectively we can plan, the more confidence we tend to gain with regards to our abilities in repeating processes, which then decreases our chances of staying in a state of chronic stress related to indecisiveness. As it relates to the unexpected condition I faced with my health as described earlier, I look back and see that I mostly took on more than I could handle. I would sometimes take on so much responsibility and sometimes not even look out for great opportunities to delegate when appropriate, to free some time to take care of other important things that I could not delegate.

As simple as it may sound now, there were times I could have trusted my family a little more to take care of the entire house, as in cleaning and making meals, and studied when necessary. However, the superwoman, great mom, and wife mentality, I realize now, led me to never want to take a break because I thought everything always had to be done in a certain perfect way, for which reason I had to always take on so much to achieve this perfection. Amidst it all, being a friendly person, saying no to some social requests sometimes I thought was unreasonable on my part, and would leave me with a sense of guilt. Now I look back and realize that there were times I could have helped others in a way that did not necessarily mean always saying 'yes'.

When I had to go through the period of difficulty with my health, I was not even able to take on all these other responsibilities that I would normally have taken on. On the flip side, I left my loved ones and friends worse off, and had to deal with the consequences of the health challenge I had suffered.

Take this from me, effective planning helps to better position you for times when you are most needed, as compared to failing to plan effectively, which has a potential of causing you to handle every situation as one that needs your attention, and many times, urgently. There are some general tips I have realized work for me repeatedly, and I believe that even though "daily to-dos" differ even on different days for the same person, you can obtain tips from my personal experiences that would help alleviate stress while you go about your day.

Do Not Overcommit

To simply describe overcommitment, it happens when you force yourself above or beyond what you are capable, or typically able to deliver or fulfill. I am not talking at all about going out of your way, or usual ability, to help someone in need of your time or service. This brings fulfillment to us as individuals.

The kind of stress we should try to fight is not just the stress that comes when we must do something needful within a short period of time. As previously described, our bodies are wired to handle that kind of stress, and able to revert to its norm in a healthy individual. Rather, it's when the stress stays prolonged for a lengthy period, that it begins to affect our health. At this unhealthy level, the body is not able to revert to its usual norm, and it begins to stay in a continual state of stress. When I talk about 'overcommitting', I'm referring to the habit of taking on too much beyond our delivery capacity or ability, and then later worrying about how we would deliver as promised.

This is one that has not been the easiest for me, and I have come to the realization that being mindful to check my calendar carefully before saying yes to any engagement is necessary of the little things as well as the big things. As a matter of fact, whether it's a big thing or seemingly small thing, all the pieces work together to make up the puzzle of your entire day, and it's necessary they fit well together.

Overcommitment can lead to being ineffective in doing what we ought to do, and in turn, contribute to chronic stress when done frequently. While at this, let me throw this in as well, as pertaining to taking on responsibilities outside of our skill sets or interests, and then worrying about how to deliver in the process. For example, accepting to decorate a venue for a friend's big party, when you know very well decorating is not an area of strength for you. This can be a source of worry for you for a friend's big party, set for the next year. On the other hand, accepting to assist someone scheduled for the decorating aspect, or even helping plan the menu, which you may know as an area of strength for you, could be a good one to accept in supporting this event. Not only would you be a better fit to deliver as promised, but you'd also be able to ensure your friend gets the best deal, and everyone is happy in the end.

Taking on responsibilities within our abilities to deliver as promised, can help us to stay effective and do more. In these choices, we would also not cause unnecessary stress to the people around us. With that said, it also means that it's sometimes very necessary for us to learn to say 'no', which can be very challenging in our daily relationships. However, it is very necessary to learn to say 'no', especially when we max out on what we can handle within any given time or given the abilities we have. There will be differences in capabilities for different people, and even for the same people within any given period or season.

Be attentive to overcommitment. 'No' is difficult to say, but sometimes it is very necessary to say, so you can do more, and of equal importance, deliver effectively whether it's work-related, or in your everyday relations. I use this to filter what I commit to, and it helps me a lot: I ask myself these simple questions:

- How long do I need to carry this request out?

- Do I have time on my schedule to accommodate it for the given period (or can I move my schedule around to accommodate this request for the given period)?

- Do I have what it takes to deliver effectively? (or can I acquire what it takes to deliver effectively given the period?)

Asking these seemingly simple questions, and looking at my given resources including time, are amazing in helping me make decisions that have to do with whether I say 'yes' to requests or not. Most importantly, the strategy of vetting requests with these questions, help me greatly in delivering effectively, while also preventing chronic stress. It also helps me to give my best not only for short periods of time but always.

More so, creating conditions of chronic stress can affect your health negatively, and can eventually also affect your performance and ability to deliver, whether at work or in your everyday relationships. Beware of overcommitment and learn to say 'no' whenever necessary.

Freedom From "Fear of The Unknown"

Fear of the unknown typically has to do with what you cannot readily influence outcomes of because it's not presently within your capacity to do so. It's also generally associated with things that would occur in the future. Future for this discussion pertains not only to the distant future but also the most immediate future, as in what will happen in let's say the next second. How easy it would be for everyone if we were able to tell what the end of a situation would mean for us. It would be easy going through the length of time it takes to get to the end, without a need to worry about the end of that situation. Not knowing what the future holds can be very stressful and can potentially turn into chronic stress if we allow anxiety to linger. This does impact our health negatively and only serves to worsen situations.

Going back to the scenario of my unexpected health interruption, I realize that I allowed my mind to be in a constant state of anxiety because I was not sure of the outcome of certain situations. For example, with my solid college science and health background, my desire to pursue a graduate school degree in business did not come easy. I already mentioned to you that I have a strong desire to be the best and reflect my best in virtually everything. So then at this stage in my life, whether it was in taking care of my family, work, or school, I had no desire to leave any of these pages in my life not meticulously attended to. For me, this meant juggling my responsibilities at a level that would help me to remain excellent in every one of these areas. As a matter of fact, my desire to go to business school was one that stemmed from a desire to help me deliver excellent services to the population I was serving. With a strong desire to continue to serve clients excellently, I went in pursuit of a degree in business. Being well equipped in the field of health to continue pursuing my passion, I realized that it was very necessary to understand the major concepts of business as well in order to deliver services with excellence. My goal was to better enhance my business knowledge and skills, so I could pursue my passion with excellence. This has always and continues to bring me a personal sense of fulfillment and joy.

You'd think I would give myself a little wiggle room, given that I was working, and had a family that needed my attention. No, I didn't. I would have done it very differently if I had to do this all over again, and still attain excellent grades without stressing myself. Hopefully, you can learn from my mistakes. I was in constant anxiety. I reflected on this experience and realized that there is absolutely nothing wrong with me being a high achiever. As a matter of fact, it is a great virtue, and I believe it is very helpful for anyone to hold dearly to such virtue.

If you are a high achiever, never beat yourself down over it. Instead, cherish it and use the proper strategies to harness greatness. There are lessons I took from this situation, which have gone a long way in helping me. I put these into practice during and after recovery and was able to finish my graduate business studies with all As, despite the health disruption. I hope you can continue to take away from some of my helpful strategies, as these will help you to achieve your goals without allowing chronic stress to set in while you're in the processes.

Stay Calm

Learning to stay calm is essential in everyone's life. For me, being calm is a key ingredient to being able to "achieve high" without the detrimental effects of chronic stress. I quickly learned that to be effective, my personal ability to stay calm, and which works immensely for me, has to be solidly rooted at all times in being mindful of leaving the outcomes of anything I do in the hands of God. That to me means, being able to trust Him totally after I have done what is within my means to accomplish my objectives. A firm trust in God diminishes anxiety and prevents chronic stress. I have learned over time to do whatever is necessary in any given situation, to positively influence outcomes, and precisely, what is humanly possible to bring about the necessary achievement that I desire. For example, as a student, I studied very well utilizing the right study habits, making sure I covered all that I was required to cover for any assignments or tests. Then again, taking any necessary extra steps that would put me ahead of the game, as in ensuring that I took any exams with good strategies. I found these to be the actions I had to personally take to attain my academic goals.

I use this simple narration to substantiate the fact that all necessary steps in the pathways to success and high achievement in any area of your life should be very well researched and followed. In other words, do not take shortcuts. Here comes the equally important step, which is often missed: after I've done all I should do, I trust God for the success of the outcome.[3] That also means I don't need to worry, knowing I have done my best.

Another major way of exercising my trust in God is in the action of learning to speak to Him (praying) throughout my day, even when it means talking to Him by asking Him questions in my heart amidst a crowd, or simply saying thank you for what He is about to do or has done in my life, at any given moment. As pertaining to trusting God, I find that memorizing the Word of God that addresses my concerns over a situation is very helpful. I try to keep The Word at the forefront of my mind, focusing and meditating on it instead of what my fears may be concerning any particular situation. For example, in my mentioned situation, I meditated on scriptures that focused on healing at a time when I was very ill. There are so many wonderful scriptures in God's word that help me to keep up with everyday challenges. Consider taking a few minutes daily to try this. There are tons of helpful resources and devotionals out there that are a great blessing. You can consider getting a good one for yourself.

At a time when I did not know what to do, I had nothing to lose in trying to trust God for healing, and it made a huge difference for me through my personal journey of finding health and healing, and it continues to work for me every day.

Trusting God will help to stir calmness in your heart and spirit and would help to prevent a state of chronic stress in your life. When feeling stressed, simply pause, say a prayer, and release the outcome of whatever situation you may be worrying about to God. A simple sentence of "God, I know you are with me and are working all this out for my good", will make a huge difference. You'll begin to see the positive effect it makes, most especially when you stay your mind on a promise from the word of God and think about it instead of worrying about an outcome of a situation you have no control over. It works amazingly well for me, and I believe it will for you also if you choose to try. Simply do your very best possible in every situation and reflect your trust in God both in your thoughts and your actions.

Be Flexible

The ability to be flexible is essential in enhancing an ability to stay calm. Many of us make plans and make them so rigid that we do not leave any room should any unexpected demands for changes occur. When things do not go as planned, we begin to worry and stress. This can lead to other forms of stress and which can potentially lead to chronic stress over time. If you are a parent, I'm sure you understand the strains that come along with accommodating the schedule of your family alongside your own. If you are the kind that strives for perfection, you also realize that you end up being in a prolonged period of stress all the time if you do not stay conscious to juggle agendas with a hint of flexibility. This used to be me and I'm sure, even if you are not a parent, you can relate to this.

The ability to be flexible has been a great asset. For example, I plan to make a little extra time on the go, to teach my kids about planning to make room for a little extra time in their own schedules. This extra time comes in handy for them whenever they have interruptions with their schedules. This is very helpful in making sure that they have enough room to meet the demands of being prompt, preferably ahead of time for anything schedule-related. For example, getting homework done ahead of time helps to prevent unnecessary potential stress that could come with starting homework when it's time to go to bed. I incorporate this same strategy in my everyday plans, and it's a win-win situation, both for myself and my family, in preventing chronic stress.

Flexibility comes in handy for me in various ways, and I mindfully think about incorporating these into whatever I do. It could be in a situation as seemingly trivial as having a plan B for dinner, in case I do not have sufficient time to deliver what I originally planned for. It could also sometimes mean, for me, making room for an hour on my schedule when planning, to complete a work-related task that would usually take about 30 minutes, during the time of my day when I expect to receive and respond to high volumes of emails. This allows me some flexibility, so that in addition to setting more realistic time frames that accommodate my typical demands, I can also deliver efficiently without the burden of continual stress. Now, pause and think about creative ways in which you could "plan to be flexible" in various areas of your life where you've found yourself constantly worrying about how to effectively complete tasks, and their related constraints of time demands. Yours may be different from mine, but I know you can easily relate to mine and I hope this stirs you into thinking about your specifics. Yes, plan to be flexible. You'll be glad you did.

Confront Your Anxiety:

Chronic anxiety can easily create chronic stress and become detrimental to your health. Let me say this again, the short-lived stress that has to do with one that your body is wired to handle, is not a problem. Typically, a healthy individual has what it takes to deal comfortably with this, and it also serves as a good boost for healthily engaging your brain and body, like I mentioned earlier. However, anxiety can become chronic when allowed to continuously prolong. Many times, this type of anxiety is linked to a "fear of the unknown in your future", and a fear of the impact of the worst occurrence, in relation to the root cause of the anxiety.

Pause, put a finger on it, and deal with the root cause head-on. This is an effective way to start "killing" anxiety before it attempts to grow into a chronic state. Be time-sensitive and precise, when it comes to finding out the root cause. These are major essentials I've found helpful with handling anxiety. My most efficient way of dealing with a potentially lingering type of anxiety is asking myself what the cause of the anxiety is, and facing it head-on, by asking what the worst situation would be if the cause prevails or assumes its worst impact on my life. For example, at the time of going through several weeks of a condition that medical doctors including specialists were unable to diagnose, I became very anxious at a certain point only to realize later that the anxiety was worsening the condition. I came to a point when I realized that I had to confront this anxiety. I asked myself what my worst fear was, and I had to answer my own question.

I thought through that and answered to myself that the worse that could happen was death. My next question was, "what next?" That was when I realized my faith in God meant so much more to me than I had ever imagined or hoped, even as relating to life after death. If you've accepted Jesus Christ as your personal Savior, then you share the same hope as I have, and should never let the fear of the unknown, even death, cause you to get into a state of chronic stress and affect your health negatively. If you haven't yet and would like to know how, read the endnotes on "Introducing My Personal Friend".

I began to encourage myself by reading more of the word of God and I knew I was assured of life after death, eternal life, which I call the "ultimate happily ever after". When that dawned on me, the scare went away, and was coupled with the trust in God that my family would always be well taken care of by Him who is taking care of me. My heart began to fill with joy, as I felt anxiety slowly go away and peace stream into my life. Anytime I had those thoughts, I began to flip them into a prayer of thanksgiving to God. I turned the sick bed into a place of communication with God.

I also read a lot of scriptures on God's will for me and my health. I realized it was God's will for me to live the full length of my days, and in good health. I would sometimes play audio formats of these scriptures while I laid down in my bed. I also believed and prayed these scriptures and prayed in faith. I trusted God and left the outcome to Him. Your absolute trust in God is an amazing way of deflecting anxiety from your emotions.

I see trusting God as leaving outcomes in the hands of someone you are certain has your best interest at heart and will ensure He works everything together to bring you the best value in the end. Many times, we worry because we try to hold on to the outcomes of situations we have no control over. More so, we get increasingly anxious in situations when we've put in the best possible actions we know how, in contributing to determining a positive outcome. Typically, at this time, we no longer have any more actions we can contribute to potentially influence the outcome the way we want it to go. Now, I believe that is where the all-knowing and well able God can be trusted to step in if we allow Him.

I remember when my kids were toddlers. There were times I would try to offer them something like a fruit, and they would hold on strongly to their toys while simultaneously attempting to grab a piece of fruit from a plate I'd serve them on. I would see them struggling to pick the fruit from the plate while holding on to their toys. Seemingly unknown to them, holding on to their toys interfered with their ability to pick the fruit from the plate, until they would let go of the toy. In this simple analogy, that is what it feels like when we try to hold on to the outcomes of situations, especially when we do not have control over these outcomes. We hold on strongly to them and their related anxieties, although we can let go and leave them in the hands of the one who has control over all situations. We can exchange this anxiety for His peace. Whether it's over the results of a game with our kids' teams, or whether or not a cake we bake will turn out perfectly like we are hoping for, we do not have control over outcomes of situations.

I cite these trivial examples to signify the fact that we do not control the outcomes of even the seemingly simple things. We can only contribute our very best to influence how any situation turns out. However, we can hold on so dearly trying to control outcomes that this can become a source of anxiety and eventually chronic stress if allowed to linger for long periods. Like the example of my kids holding on to toys in their hands while also trying to grab slices of fruit from a plate, it would be very difficult to accept the fact that God holds the outcome, and trust Him, if we mentally position ourselves to be the sole determinants of outcomes. In this state, we hold on rigidly to those thoughts along with the consequential anxieties that come with making sure they turn out just the way we want them to. A major part of trusting God can be compared to letting go of your outcomes-related fears and anxieties, releasing these to Him, trusting Him as you position yourself to receive His best. This can bring you so much peace because you stop worrying about the outcome, while also being hopeful you'd have the best possible outcome. This is because you have totally given that charge to someone who not only cares about you but is also working all things for your good. When you win, He wins too! Trusting God worked and continues to work wonders for me, and I believe it will for you also.

As I began to trust God through these simple steps with my health, suddenly after a couple of months of continuously battling with chronic anxiety through the period of my health struggles, the tables turned around. I watched my sick bed begin to turn slowly around into a place of healing. I began to gradually experience strength in my body, the swelling in my lymph nodes resolved at an equally gradual pace until I was able to function at my normal capacity. I was then able to resume involvement with some of the things I loved to do, as in participating in activities with my family and friends.

It was gradual but sure worth the wait, and worth putting in the effort in battling anxiety, and of course, chronic stress. This personal experience is a great support of the fact that taking good care of your spiritual health, does have a significant impact on your mental and emotional health which ultimately impacts your physical health. I am a living proof of this.

It's no wonder there is a cry for the need of a holistic approach to healthcare, where not only the body is taken care of, but where things are done to incorporate care of the spirit and the mind. Very truly, these domains interact with each other to impact the whole health of an individual, as seen in some of the possible effects of anxiety on the body, as it turns into chronic stress. Today, there are many ways by which people take care of their bodies spiritually.

For me, I can tell you what has been special about choosing to go the way of Jesus Christ. This is the fact that I have answers not only to take care of my now or present anxieties and fears, but I have the assurance of a "happily ever after" (eternal life), even after death. This only serves to further put to rest my greatest fear of the unknown, life after death. That makes a huge difference for me, and I believe it can for you also if you choose to accept Jesus as your personal Lord and Savior if you haven't already done so. Great thing, He will help you deal with anxiety also.

I must say that the major causes of anxiety can be in any format that connects to your fear of the unknown. Sometimes, something like not knowing what would happen to you next as you witness your colleagues being fired from work could stir chronic anxiety in you. As I mentioned earlier, the best way I've found to deal with fear of the unknown is to confront it head-on with personal questions about what the worst, extreme, situations could possibly be.

Next, answering these questions and then making sure you've put in place measures that would help you to boldly face these extreme situations should they occur, is of significant help. Doing this would help alleviate the anxiety, from its root cause. For example, in the firing situation, find a new job, while adjusting current spending to accommodate the loss of a job. This would be a good plan to put in place. The plan will help you to start saving also if you are not already doing so.

Many times, the things we stress about or are fearful of, never even happen. Yet, many are affected by and suffer more so from the stress of the possible occurrence than from the actual occurrence of the situation. Be vigilant, deal with anxiety head-on! Do what it takes to prevent it from lingering.

The World Health Organization defines health as a state of absolute physical, mental and social well-being and not just the absence of disease or illness.[4] I can't say this enough: your mental and emotional states of health matter and they influence your physical health. Anxiety contributes immensely to upsetting your body and your overall health. Beware of it and nick it before it daringly tries to nick you. Always keep in mind the fact that your strong ability to deal effectively with those little stressful situations, can help prevent advancement into a state of chronic stress within your body. Use these strategies to your advantage!

Turn Up Your Game!

There are other seemingly minor but very important things I have learned to do all through my day that also help me to stay on top of preventing a creep of chronic stress, while also using some of my major strategies previously described. An important key is, stay vigilant, and do this by the minute, daily! With the right tactics in place, you can turn up the entire "game" of keeping your body in great health.

Did you know that what you eat does affect the state of your body, including your emotional and mental health? It really does! Processed and refined carbohydrates like candies, doughnuts, etc. have a way of delivering sugar quickly to the body. These refined carbohydrates have little to no fiber and can deliver sugar so quickly to your bloodstream that they are typically able to rapidly increase blood sugar levels outside your normal desired ranges. This will give your body more work to do in terms of keeping up with regulating the high levels of sugar "flood" into the bloodstream during those times.

This tires your body out. With a quick influx of large volumes of sugar to the bloodstream from eating these refined carbohydrates, the body must do the job of storing some of the sugar in certain organs. The body must also perform major functions necessary to keep the levels of sugar in the bloodstream within an acceptable range while trying to store some of the excess sugar. After working so hard to keep the high levels of sugar in check, this can potentially lead to a period of stress, following the period of a sugar rush. In contrast, carbohydrates from their unprocessed/unrefined states typically have some fiber and can steadily go through the digestive process, working "gently" over a period of time to keep your blood sugar levels within a good range without "overwhelming" it with a quick high-level of influx.

Hungry and craving something sweet? Consider choosing a banana over candies. High fiber-containing foods keep your stomach full longer. Eating foods containing high amounts of fiber can prevent excessive eating along with its consequence of unnecessary weight gain for most people. This is even more beneficial when coupled with a good source of healthy proteins and other vegetables.

Additionally, processed carbohydrates tend to get you into a cycle of frequent cravings for them and can keep you eating lots of them. The good thing is, you can break this cycle by simply making a choice to overlook them for a few days. Like a bad habit, if done consistently for about three weeks, you'll be in control. Beyond that time, you get to be the boss and maintain control by choosing to eat them occasionally, solely at your discretion. With you deciding to be in control, you can curb your cravings for them.

Are you thinking of switching from artificial sweeteners and other sugar substitutes? There are lots of great natural alternatives to sugar like honey and many others. However, there are also lots of artificially manufactured sugar substitutes and processed foods that contain components which can interfere with the normal pathways of metabolism. These can end up causing more harm to the body than you can possibly think of. For example, aspartame, a popular substitute for sugar, has been found to incite various health conditions including headaches, mood disorders, inclusive of depression.[5,6] Foods with low calories may not always be healthy. Read ingredient labels!

Additionally, some of these substances are toxic to the body and can also potentially accumulate over time within, causing damage to body cells. It's no wonder some of these have been found to be cancer-causing. My goal is for you to remember the major reasons to stay away from some of these. Let me tell you personally, that I would choose real sugar any day over artificial sweeteners. The most important thing to remember is to consume sugar in small quantities when at all, as this would help you to stay low on sugar consumption, which is a great health goal. Reading labels when you go shopping, can help you to enjoy great emotional, mental, and physical health.

Excessively consuming deep-fried foods can also impact your mood negatively and lead to chronic stress. Deep-fried foods are typically loaded with trans-fat, which has been linked to causes of depression.[7] Do you remember the ability of trans-fat to clog arteries as mentioned in Chapter 4? This can potentially decrease blood flow to the brain and affect moods also. Consider limiting and keeping the consumption of deep-fried foods very minimal on your menu.

High consumption of processed foods and "junk" like we term it, as in eating high amounts of fast foods in terms of both quantities and frequency, can be dangerous to your health. In addition to causing many health problems, as in some of those previously mentioned in the broad sense, the potentially negative effect of these on the body's mental state of health should be considered when making choices. Frequency and amounts of consumption matters. Consider limiting both quantity and frequency of consumption of these foods, and you'd be amazed at the difference this little step could make in your mental health and mood.

Most processed foods are also high in sodium. This can negatively affect your body's overall performance in many ways when consumed in high amounts. Various metabolic and functional pathways can be affected, including the body's blood pressure function as well as functional pathways within the neurological system. This can result in a negative impact on the body's mental health as well. In fact, high frequency of fast food consumption has been linked to a high incidence of depression in midlife women.[8]

Since nutrients from food contribute immensely to the formation of bodily components both in structure and function inclusive of cells, hormones, etc., it is no wonder that intake of substances that interfere with pathways of formation of these bodily components also interfere with the body's general state of health. Keep in mind, "junk in, junk out". More importantly to take out, "healthy in, healthy out".

High levels of caffeine consumption have been linked to anxiety, stress, and negative effects on mental health.[9, 10] Here comes another helpful concept, the *concept of moderation.* In the use of this concept, it's important to know the occasional benefits of taking an action, as well as its downside with higher frequency. With this knowledge, find your *perfect personal frequency*, where you'd obtain benefits without the downside. This *personal perfect frequency* would be different for each individual, and you'd need to observe yourself to find yours. In the application of the *concept of moderation*, I introduce variable uses, as in that of *purposeful moderation*. In *purposeful moderation*, purposefully cap this action below your *perfect personal frequency* whenever you take this action. I discuss lots of helpful strategies as to how to use *moderation* to the advantage of your health throughout the book. With this in mind, let me mention that some studies have shown health benefits in consuming limited daily quantities of caffeine in certain groups of healthy adult populations. Researching both sides of the story and from my personal experience, I like to stay within the limits of the *concept of purposeful moderation*. In application, rarely and or occasionally consuming caffeine with *personal perfect frequency* in mind is helpful. This is because for certain individuals, consuming limited quantities, is okay. "Listen" to your body's responses to varying amounts of caffeine consumption, and I believe it will tell you exactly what your personal amounts in the practice of the *concept of moderation* should be.

Rare and or occasional consumption is a great way to keep away from the excesses that affect so many people. I say so because for some people, taking caffeine initially helps them to stay highly alert and awake to complete certain tasks whether it's work-related or study-related. Over time, caffeine and sugar can get addictive if you become dependent on it. At that level of dependency, many people begin to increase the quantities they consume just to obtain the same effects they started off with.

At the same time of having large amounts of caffeine in the body with possible negative side effects, the impact from staying alert and awake over long periods of time break the necessary ability of the body to calm down, rest, and "catch its breath". It's no wonder that in some people, this progresses into nervousness. The nervousness when prolonged can advance to become a significant source of chronic stress, affecting the body's mental state of health. Do you see how this prolonged period of "alertness" can deprive the body of needed rest, with a potential of creating a state of "chronic stress"? Always remember when it comes to preventing chronic stress, that periods of "intermittent rest" is necessary for good health.

Here's a helpful tip: stay away from resorting to caffeine as a means of helping you to stay awake and alert for long periods. It's potential negative latent effect especially on your mental, and eventually your physical health may not be worth the try, not to mention its potentially addictive effects. Consider joining the occasional consumption group in minimal quantities when at all possible. My advice, especially to high school and college students, do not resort to coffee as an aid for learning, in keeping you alert. It may seem attractive initially but has a great potential of negatively affecting your state of mind and health in the long run. It's also potentially addictive. Limiting it to occasional consumption in small quantities not only keeps you in control over it, but will keep you away from the long-term potentially negative side effects. Adults will benefit from this advice as well. It is possible for you to train your body to rest when needed and awaken to work or study when you need to. Although difficult to do sometimes, once you try to stay in charge a few times, you'll find it worth the try. If I can do this, you can also. Remember also, that planning your time effectively will help you to avoid the need to frequently stay awake for prolonged hours, trying to meet deadlines. It is possible to stay on top of your daily demands if you plan effectively.

This connects to the subject of alcohol, one that has a strong ability to heavily affect the body's mental state. It simply depresses the central nervous system. One can easily tell from the erratic behavior displayed by people when under the influence, without me going into excessive detail. The tricky aspect of drinking alcohol is the fact that there is a very fine line between switching from what people would describe as tolerable quantities (different for different people), to when its "toxicity" overpowers you. This fine line is not easy to detect, and for the sake of great health, it is helpful to stay away from it. I personally choose to stay completely away from it and highly recommend this to loved ones and friends. It is very addictive for people who frequently get overpowered by a high consumption. This can also contribute heavily to chronic stress in individuals who fall prey to it.

I hope the broad discussion of some of the foods that influence mental health and moods will be helpful to you when making food choices that impact your health. Simply put, these foods have a great potential of contributing immensely to causing a state of chronic stress in the body. In fact, people battling depression are encouraged to avoid refined sugar, artificial sweeteners, processed foods, hydrogenated oils, high sodium containing foods, caffeine, and alcohol when at all possible.[11] These foods are key players and have a strong ability to negatively affect the mental state of health.

In as much as it is good to watch out for foods that can negatively impact your mental and emotional state of health and limit consumption of them, ending there would not be enough as pertaining to taking care of the state of your mental health. It is equally important to deliberately look out for, and incorporate foods into your diet, that positively affect your mental state of health.

Do you remember the phrase "gut feeling"? As ridiculous as it sounds, there is truly an amazing literal relationship between your gut and your feelings. And yes, aspects of your feelings do have a heavy connection to your gut, and if you pay attention to what goes into your gut in the literal sense, you can also have a healthier impact on your everyday moods and feelings. The literal analysis of this phrase is as true as the implicative use of what we know the actual meaning to be.

This reminds me of an "aha" moment I had during an embryology class in my undergraduate Biology Study. I remember one time when I was extensively studying how a baby (at a time when it's not yet even recognized as a human) after conception in its very early stages develops (The study of embryology). I very well remember reading about how a specific ball of cells together at a certain time during this embryo formation, divide and have a part of the ball of cells separate from the original whole to form major components of the brain and spinal cord (The Central Nervous System). The remaining components from this ball of cells then proceed to form components of the gut (The Enteric Nervous System), with the vagus nerve linking the brain and the gut.

The vagus nerve is a portion of the involuntary nervous system. It works to stimulate major actions of the body where your will or your ability to deliberately control things is not involved. Some involuntary actions include digestion of the food you eat, and the beating of your heart, to mention a couple. During this time of study, the "lights" turned on for me, as I thought I had a good understanding of the term "gut feeling" I realized that part of the central nervous system (which includes the brain) has something at the beginning of formation of the embryo to do with portions of the gut, as they originate from the same initial ball of cells. Not to go into extensive detail, I highlighted this to state that there must still be a reason for us to remember how the brain and the gut are linked and relate, even from fetal formation, at the time when we began formation in the womb.

A major substance (neurotransmitter) called serotonin, which mediates a wide range of physiological functions within the body, is also known to play a mood-enhancing role. Close to 90% of serotonin is produced in the gut and platelets of the blood, while the amounts used by the brain is produced by the brain. Serotonin has been known to play a role in most types of behaviors, including emotional, appetite regulation, cognition, and many others.[12]

It is no wonder a major way of treating depression medically, relies heavily on medications collectively containing SSRIs (selective serotonin reuptake inhibitors), which work by preventing the brain's reabsorption of the serotonin it produces. This makes serotonin widely available in the body to carry out essential functions, as in mood enhancement. You may be familiar with some of these drugs such as Prozac, Paxil, Zoloft, to name a few[13], typically prescribed by physicians in treating certain mood disorders like depression. The state of your body's emotion has a close link and relationship with the state of your mental health.

To help make an easy connection in this discussion, I will occasionally refer to mental health as "head health". The state of health of your gut tends to affect your emotional health and wellbeing, both in the literal sense as well as figuratively. Now, figuratively, when I mentioned "gut feeling", I said so to illustrate the fact that occasionally, everyone may have some feelings which may appear to originate from the "gut" but are still able to influence the brain to make the right decisions in certain instances. For many of us, you know these feelings tend to be ones you don't just ignore.

My children simply call it "the little siren": when you have that feeling something may not be right, but do not have literal backing from your "head" in terms of explanation to support that feeling. Under such circumstances, you still know there is some seemingly "remote" part of your brain that supports what you're feeling. Hopefully, my little lesson from my embryology class helps you to understand that the gut and central nervous system do have some relationship with each other, that originated during formation in your mother's womb. If one part, the brain, now literally "thinks", then the other that does not literally think (the gut) may indirectly have some inherent ability to "think", if they originated from the same "parent", the initial ball of cells I mentioned.

Taking it a step further, can I tell you in literal terms also, that what you eat affects the condition of your mental health? From all the different explanations I have given, I'm sure you deeply understand that if you want a healthy mental and emotional state of health, you should also pay attention to what you eat. Be mindful of your "gut health" (what you eat), as it affects your "head health", your emotions, and your overall wellbeing.

Having discussed the need to put the right foods in your body even as it relates to the state of your mental and emotional health, I believe a large portion of my goal in this section has been achieved. I'll go ahead with broad discussions that will help you to put this concept into practice. Connecting some ideas from some of our previous discussions, you'll realize that an important rule of the thumb is to eat highly nutritious foods, keeping the consumption of deep-fried and processed foods to a minimum. Eating a wide variety of foods rich in color (bright and dark alike) will help you to consume a lot of the nutrients that are amazing mood enhancers.

Maintaining great gut health is essential for mood enhancement. In as much as we talk a lot about germs (pathogens) that try to invade the body and cause disease, we would be doing ourselves a great disservice if we did not understand also, that there are good bacteria, as I'll call them, that live in our bodies and help us carry out processes that keep us in good shape. The gut (digestive system) is a major hub for these good bacteria. All the way from our mouths through our intestines, these good bacteria help to break down the foods we eat into forms that the body can absorb well. This helps to ensure that we have nutrients getting into our bloodstream and going through to various parts of our bodies to help in carrying out major bodily functions.

Without going into extensive detail, let me mention that there are some good bacteria that help not only with the digestion of the foods we eat, but also help with the production of some key vitamins. Good bacteria also aid in fighting certain harmful bacteria that attempt to invade the body and cause disease. A major and quick way of increasing the amounts of good bacteria in the gut is by eating fermented foods in healthy quantities while maintaining an ability to make good choices from the wide varieties out there. Being mindful of factors like high sodium content in certain foods, as well as artificial additives such as artificial sweeteners, is helpful to keep in mind when shopping for fermented foods. With this guide in mind, it would be easier to make great choices whether it's from dairy (as in your yogurts, etc.), vegetables, or any other sources of foods that are fermented. Keep in mind, a goal of eating with the most benefits to your health at heart is essential. I carefully stated this because many times I have seen people making choices of food with only one goal in mind (such as getting good bacteria from fermented foods), while ignoring any potential health-related red flags (such as dangerous additives and preservatives) that may come along with some of these foods.

My aim is to provide a broad picture of a better overall understanding so you are empowered to make your best choices when it comes down to making your preferred picks in actual practice. Some people choose to use probiotics whether it's recommended by their physician, or they pick them while grocery shopping, to help make available good bacteria in their guts. It is very possible to get what you need in terms of good flora by making the right food picks. However, if you ever need to go the route of probiotics, be sure to check with your physician, especially if you have any health concerns. Certain good bacteria in your gut help with proper digestion so that when you eat, you also have the nutrients made available to various parts of your body through your bloodstream. Available nutrients help you to properly carry out major bodily functions. If this process goes well through the right series of actions, it in turn positively affects the state of your mental and emotional health.

Furthermore, there are foods that have been found to enhance moods. Omega-3 fatty acid-rich foods are great mood-enhancers and have even been noted to improve negative mood symptoms in certain depressive individuals. Nuts, with a popular one being walnut, are generally rich in omega-3. Fish is also generally a rich source, especially those that abound with healthy oils, such as salmon, sardines, etc. Various sources of plant foods are rich in omega 3 oils, such as those from flaxseed, chia seed, just to name a few. Whole grains also tend to be rich in omega 6 and 3 fatty acids. This is a major reason why it's important to choose whole grain bread any day over plain white flour bread. The little choices you make everyday matter and can go a long way in enhancing your mood and health. Keep in mind these foods rich in healthy oils will also work to decrease your body's levels of bad fats and increase your levels of good fats. They work closely together to manage your body's total cholesterol, as well as heart and brain health. Do you see a clear example showing the interdependence of the body's systems on each other beautifully depicted here again?

Choices of whole grains also help to contribute to your body's daily requirement of fiber, very necessary to provide "bulk" to move the food you eat along in your digestive tract. This helps to foster proper digestion and elimination, which eventually also contributes immensely to your overall state of health. While fiber provides this "bulk" during digestion to move food along the digestive tract by a mechanism called peristaltic movements, it also helps to prevent your body from keeping remnants from digested foods for long periods in your colon. These peristaltic movements are an involuntary contraction and relaxation of the muscles of the intestines, that provide a wave-like motion, moving food along the tract during digestion. Fiber provides the necessary "bulk" that helps to make this motion effective.

There are several other factors that can interfere with peristalsis, although an inadequate intake of fiber is a common but often overlooked one. Insufficient daily intake of fiber can deprive the body of carrying out this peristaltic function efficiently, by preventing the successful movement of food along the tracts for proper digestion. Some days, meeting that requirement may be challenging. However, even on those days, you can aim at simply eating an apple if possible or making every effort to get immediately back on track, the subsequent days. Keeping digestive remnants for long periods in the gut has a huge possibility of increasing the chances of the body absorbing unwanted "stuff" inclusive of possible toxins. These non-moving digestive remnants can also cause feelings of bloating and discomfort. This can negatively affect the body's mental state of health as well.

Do you know anyone who went through a process of recovery from surgery or an illness? Do you remember some of the major things their healthcare team was interested in keeping track of? I'm sure they asked for signs that indicated there was proper movement along the digestive tract. They might have asked questions about gas or bowel movement. The little choices you make to have a healthy state of gut and mental health, can go a long way to also help in other intertwined areas of your health. Those little choices matter and can contribute greatly to help boost your overall health.

Low levels of iron have been greatly associated with low cognitive function. Foods that are rich in iron are great mood boosters. This is because iron helps with the adequate formation of red blood cells that help with the circulation of oxygen and essential nutrients around the body. Healthy levels of iron help to make oxygen and essential nutrients available to the brain, to boost its function.

Conditions that affect circulation can also typically affect cognition. In some people, problems with cognition can be seen in the form of them showing signs of confusion, as pertaining to the subject of this discussion. Cognition-related issues resulting from poor circulation can stimulate or even worsen mood disorders in some people with existing depressive conditions. Bear in mind that this is only an example of a possible cause or agitation in some instances, of these disorders. There are tons of other possible causes of mood disorders, including hormonal imbalances and much more, beyond the scope of our current discussion.

My focus at this point, is on the importance of using potential benefits from our everyday choices of foods, to naturally enhance our health. Choosing the right foods can help your body maintain and, in certain instances, regain health, as it was in my situation. Some foods which are rich in iron, are also rich in zinc. Zinc is a mineral well known for its ability to boost immune health. These foods include your red meats like beef, as well as your dark poultry meats. Eating lean portions from a variety of these about 3-4 times interspersed within your week can go a long way to ensure you have a good supply of these essential nutrients. My personal preference is keeping beef minimal, with a broad picture of my overall nutritional intake in proper perspective. I try to be creative with getting my daily iron intake. Be sure to look out for helpful tips in Chapters 20 & 25 that will empower you to stay in control as well with this subject. Knowing the sources of iron and the relative quantities they provide to the body is a great way to stay on top of your daily iron intake.

There are other ways by which you can gain some of these nutrients, as from your green leafy vegetables, etc. The key is, be attentive to include a wide variety of healthy picks in your diet, ensuring adequate amounts of foods containing some of these essential nutrients. Sometimes, I tend to think that some of what we attribute to hormonal imbalance-related mood swings in women, very real and true, many times have significant ties also to inadequate intake of nutrient-rich foods that can enhance moods and impact hormonal levels in the body.

My personal observation is that many women tend to focus on little aspects of their health and take on certain extreme diet modifications without taking into consideration the impact some of these diets would make on their overall health. Whether it's for weight loss or a specific health condition, it's important to understand what you do and the impact it has on your overall health. This is also true for men. I understand the impact of allergies when present, or restrictions on certain foods that have adverse effects on certain individuals, as in examples related to a possible interaction with a prescription medication. I address some myths related to foods in the latter part of the book.

Be open to eating a variety, with a good understanding of what matters most, and what should be consumed in minimal quantities. Your wide variety of beans and soy are a good source of zinc also. Various aspects of brain function and mood have been positively enhanced in pre-menopausal women, when provided with an increased intake of iron and zinc.[14]

As a mother with growing kids, I realize that not only is paying attention to my diet important, but it is of equal importance in the life of every member of my family. How many times do we see children, youth, and young adults showing unusual patterns in their moods and behavior, and tend to quickly attribute names of familiar diagnoses to these behavior patterns, without first analyzing what they are eating? Do not overlook the fact that what you eat can significantly affect the levels of hormonal production in your body, and consequentially how you feel.

You are either boosting your health by the choices of what you put in your stomach, or negatively impacting your health by these same choices of food. I understand that many other choices can affect health, some of which no one has control over. However, I also understand you have control over the choices of food you eat. Why not use this to your advantage?

If you are a teenager or young adult reading this book, I must commend you for making the choice to read it because it will help you to gain a strong overall foundation that will equip you to make healthier choices and enjoy your life, not only now but in the many years ahead of you. In addition to some of the major categories of mood-boosting foods discussed, I must mention that dark chocolate has been noted as one that has high antioxidant properties.[15] Dark chocolate has high levels of polyphenols, a group of micronutrients in certain foods, that afford them high antioxidant properties. It has been shown to be a great mood enhancer as well as one that also has great benefits to the health of the heart. As previously discussed, be sure to keep in mind sugar and other additives in your choices of dark chocolate, and of course, go for choices in its purest form as much as possible. Like I always say, if I must eat candy, at least, let my dark chocolate choice count toward a better cause.

With this broad understanding, there is a wide range of healthy mood-boosting foods to choose from. Explore, and keep in mind, the wider the variety of healthy picks you make, the better it is for enhancing your overall state of health. Remember to explore a wide variety of colors of fruits and vegetables, especially keeping in mind some of the broad concepts discussed. Also, try to keep junk minimal.

CHAPTER SEVEN

Let The Butterflies Loose

Making plans to unwind while deliberately engaging in activities that help release endorphins in your brain is vital to your health and wellness.

Have you ever questioned if you could ever truly feel good most times? Let me dare to tell you that this can be so for you if you purposely try to focus on working on it. And guess what? There are hormones that enhance this process which in turn can positively enhance your health. I call these hormones the "feel good hormones". As simple as the name I've given this may sound, these hormones are very essential to boosting your immune health. Of equal significance is the fact that it takes very simple bodily actions, although usually easily overlooked, to secrete these hormones and put them to work. These actions are what I equate to "letting the butterflies loose". The "feel good hormones" that are released when the "butterflies are let loose", can go a long way to fight the onset of chronic stress while boosting your immune health in the process. I discuss these "feel good hormones" with tips on how you can deliberately let the "butterflies" loose to release their action.

Let me take you back to my analogy of putting out fires by using means that would cut the fire's access to oxygen, to prevent it from continual burning (from Chapter 4). It's important to add here, that there are various other means of stopping fires from continual burning, right in their tracks. There are other lines of fire extinguishers known as the stored pressure fire extinguishers. These are most commonly found in industrial facilities and they use carbon dioxide as a means of extinguishing fires.[1] Carbon dioxide, unlike oxygen, simply "kills" fires, and does not help to keep the burning process going. It does the opposite of what oxygen does. There is also the method of using water by firemen as a means of putting out fires at certain times. Again, water does not promote the burning of fires. It does the opposite. What am I trying to say? Like the many options available that can help to put out fires, there are also various other ways besides what we eat, that may simply improve our feelings of happiness and stir up the secretion of good hormones that can boost our immune health. These options can act as great stress relievers.

Have you heard this saying: "Laughter is as good as medicine"? Laughter can stimulate a release of hormones called endorphins, which I refer to as the "feel good hormones". This release of endorphins, in turn, can stir up a feeling of happiness within us. Endorphins can even produce a pain killing effect, by interacting with your brain receptors responsible for regulating your levels of pain perception. Yes, your smile could be that powerful in boosting your health!

A release of these endorphins is triggered when your facial muscles are composed in a way that simulates that of laughter, or even a smile. The next time you are tempted to hold back a smile because you think it only benefits the receiver, remember you also gain from that kind act. Dare to give that smile. Your body deserves that benefit.

There are days when mastering a smile to give someone may seem like something a little too difficult for you to do because of what you may personally be going through. I understand those days. However, I would dare to say that even on those days, pluck up the courage to still pull through with those smiles and try to make the day of the people you come into contact with beautiful. While you do that, you also boost a release of endorphins in your body, that can act as a potent stress reliever and help you to feel good.

The action of endorphins is very opposite that of cortisol. Keep in mind the fact that cortisol is a major hormone, that gets busy in action, helping your body to combat some of the potentially negative effects, when you feel stressed. Endorphins, on the other hand, are released to boost your feelings of happiness when they are stimulated into action. Up those endorphins, with something as simple as a smile. Furthermore, you can never go wrong with filling your mind with positive thoughts, one that also positions you for secretion of endorphins and creates a cycle of good feeling. This is a major antidote to stress.

To enhance the production of endorphins, find and make time to enjoy some of the activities that make you happy some time throughout your day, even if it's only for five minutes. Some of my favorites include taking a walk, talking, and laughing with friends and or family, watching a comedy together with them, or by myself, reading a good book, my favorite of which is the Bible. You can easily create your favorite set of activities also if you do not already have those in place. It is very important to plan for moments in your day to simply unwind.

Focus on activities you enjoy that would up your levels of the "feel-good hormones" (endorphins). If you haven't yet, consider finding this set from the many activities you currently have that you enjoy doing, and rotate to find a good balance.

While varying your activities, keep in mind the fact that exercising can help you to "kill multiple birds with one stone". By that, I mean in addition to all the other benefits of it, exercising can also help your body to secrete endorphins. In planning unwinding activities, I highly recommend putting activities that involve some forms of exercising as priority on your list. Even at work, utilize your time effectively, and include purposefully planning to take your lunch breaks. Taking your planned breaks can help you to stay even more productive. Being too busy to take necessary breaks can be counterproductive to being effective. Making plans to unwind, while deliberately engaging in activities that help release endorphins in your brain will help you feel good. These are great ways of preventing chronic stress and boosting your immune and overall health.

After going through the challenge with my health, I realized how important it is to consciously put some of these stress-relieving strategies into action. I've found that doing this helps me stay in better shape in terms of my mental health. I also think about my thoughts, so I can steer myself to focus on positive, health-boosting thoughts. Preventing chronic stress is very vital, and you can do it by utilizing some of these strategies to your advantage. Now, sit back, and be intentional in letting the "butterflies" loose. Your goal is to be deliberate in doing this daily via the simple actions you already love to perform.

CHAPTER EIGHT

Your Swimming Pool:
Make It A Fabulous One!

*All it takes is the courage to decide,
and the perseverance to pursue change
in the right direction!*

I f you have a swimming pool in your home, you may have an
idea of the several tasks involved in maintaining a pool. For
this discussion, I'll focus on the task of maintaining the PH
of your pool's water. In this example, the PH has to do with the
acidity or alkalinity of the pool. Here comes my connection: I
compare the water in the pool to the blood in our bodies, which
is an important red-colored liquid in the arteries of our body
that carries oxygen and nutrients to the various tissues of the
body. Blood also takes carbon dioxide and "wastes" away from
the tissues to the lungs and other parts of the body, where the
"exchanges" and "recycles" for renewal occur. In providing a simple description, let me mention that blood is made up of various
components which are highly vital to the maintenance of our

bodily functions. As you may have guessed by now from my introductory analogy, the "house" I'm referring to, is your body.

In the case of the swimming pool, the PH must be just right, for anyone who uses the pool to obtain potential benefits. A slightly basic PH, not too distant from neutral is recommended when it comes to swimming pools, with many maintaining a PH typically between 7.2 to 7.5. Keep in mind, 7 is a neutral reference point when it comes to PH measurements. Numbers above 7 head in the direction of alkalinity, and below 7 head in the direction of acidity. One of the major goals when formulating an ideal swimming pool PH is getting it to be as close as possible to the PH of the mucous membranes and the eyes of human users who will swim in it. This PH tries to ensure that swimming conditions are comfortable and safe for users, while at the same time ensuring that swimming pool components function effectively for their targeted use. Hence, in striving for pool maintenance, one of the major goals is to keep the water in the pool within this tight range of targeted PH levels.

Extreme conditions outside of the target range, whether alkalinity or acidity, can stir up chemical reactions which can cause potential dangers. For example, a highly acidic environmental pool condition could stimulate chemical reactions in metallic components of the pool, when they are present. This can lead to the production of chemical by-products which could pose potential harm to the skin of swimmers. A highly alkaline environment on the flip side can potentially stimulate reaction in plumbing components, making the pool cloudy and creating an unfavorable condition for swimmers. Furthermore, in a highly acidic environment, the chlorine added to the water to kill bad bugs (pathogens) would disperse quickly. The chlorine would also not do its job very well in a highly alkaline environment. There are times when the PH levels would attempt to get out of the targeted ideal range because of the various activities performed in the water by users. However, because of the need to maintain the targeted range to ensure maximum performance always, chemicals are added as needed to keep up with the desired levels of PH for the water.

Do you see how this analogy could relate to the blood in our bodies? Keep in mind that the blood is always busy performing its activities of nourishing our tissues as it takes nutrients and oxygen to them, while also taking carbon dioxide and wastes away from them. Like the scenario of the pool, the various activities carried about by the blood can cause it to fall out of its desired PH range, most especially in a diseased state.

In a normal healthy individual, the body has mechanisms in place that tightly regulate the blood's PH based on interactions from various systems of the body. Therefore, it's typically very rare for the blood to remain outside of its normal PH for a long time without the body putting in hard work to bring it back to normal. There are times when we put so much burden on the blood via our various activities, whether knowingly, as from eating excessive unhealthy foods, or unknowingly, as from our skin's excessive absorption of potentially harmful substances and irritants from the environment. Under most circumstances, the blood perseveres in doing its job tirelessly, unless, we put undue "stress" on an organ that feeds into this process by any chance, and the organ slows or breaks down in function. This organ "malfunction" can eventually also affect the blood's performance in carrying out its essential role.

Many times, organs involved in this process are interconnected to each other by their function. For example, you might have heard about how a dysfunction in the liver can negatively impact the liver in its ability to rid the body's "wastes" that are produced as byproducts of metabolic functions within the body. These "wastes" are carried from tissues into the bloodstream as the blood circulates nutrients and other essentials for the body's function. The liver helps to break down some of these "wastes" and helps to "detoxify" the body.

In taking care of their patients, most physicians are very particular about monitoring liver function via blood test results, especially if they are planning on prescribing medications that demand an active involvement of the liver. In fact, there are certain instances related to administering certain medications that nurses have been trained to be careful in checking test results related to liver function before administering those. This can also occur for many other organs in the body, however, I am focusing on the liver because of its connection regarding to our discussion.

With the image of how the swimming pool needs to maintain its ideal PH to effectively perform all the functions, necessary for its very existence, so does the human body. It is interesting to mention that the ideal, normal PH of blood in the body's arteries is 7.4. From the swimming pool example, you know that this is a slightly alkaline environment. Going extremely below 7.4 will create an acidic environment and going extremely above 7.4 will make the environment highly alkaline.

In a healthy individual, the body has systems in place that help it to keep the blood within this slightly alkaline range, usually between 7.3 to 7.45. The body tries via various means to maintain an ideal state within its various interconnected systems, no matter what may be happening around it. The body does this through a process called homeostasis. This homeostasis is an ability of the body to seek and maintain a stable internal condition when dealing with changes in its external environment. For the focus of this discussion, maintaining a targeted range of PH in its blood.

The blood is a vital component of the circulatory system of the body. Do you remember that a major function of the blood is carrying oxygen and nutrients to the various tissues in the body, while also carrying carbon dioxide and "wastes" away from these tissues, for excretion? For the blood to effectively do its job, the body tries to perform various other functions to help it to maintain its ideal PH. Like the swimming pool maintenance person, our job is to provide the body with the nutrients, necessary for it to maintain this ideal, slightly alkaline environment.

I will not go into extreme details biologically as to how all this is done. However, I find it very necessary to paint this broad picture, so you will be able to mentally connect to its importance. Stay in control of giving your body what it needs to maintain this slightly alkaline environment within your blood, as in the ideal pool PH which helps the pool to retain chlorine necessary to rid itself of pathogens.

It is very important to empower your body to carry out functions, necessary to help it maintain its ideal PH. You'll realize that there are many simple foods that contain potent nutritious substances that can help you to do just that. One of my favorites is the juice from lemons. They are amazing! You'll find out why in Chapter 16.

The kidneys, the respiratory system, and many other organs and systems within the body, carry out various functional processes to help in maintaining the blood's ideal PH. Let me use a simple analogy that will help to create a broad mental picture of this buffering system within the body. Imagine mixing hot water (maybe the highly alkaline state), and cold water (maybe the highly acidic state) to create lukewarm water for you to take a shower. When you want an ideal temperature in let's say, water from your bathtub, you'd adjust the levels of hot or cold water, in the direction of how you want it until you reach your ideal temperature goal. It's a comparable process the body carries out to help the blood to maintain its ideal PH.

The kidney is a major organ that helps in the process, usually, the value of the kidney's effect realized over many hours as compared to that of the respiratory system and that of proteins and other chemical buffers which have their effects realized relatively more quickly. The body depends on both the quick actors and the relatively slow actors in helping the blood to stay within the ideal PH range. One of the simplest things we can do on our part is to provide the body with nutrients that can help it maintain this ideal PH.

The body's functions are intricately interconnected. Putting the "right" things into our digestive system is a major way by which we can help empower the body to get what it needs to effectively do what it needs to do. This is one major area that I believe God has placed within our capabilities when it comes to taking care of our bodies. It is very helpful to always ask God for wisdom, and the grace to be able to do that.

To further explain how intricately the systems and functions of our bodies are interconnected and interdependent of each other, let me mention that an ideal PH is necessary for oxygen to be adequately "dissolved" in the blood, as well as nutrients, to be efficiently carried to the various tissues. Again, using the lukewarm water analogy, amidst other factors, a slightly elevated, above room temperature glass of water, would dissolve a cube of sugar better than water at room temperature, or even one that has been chilled in a refrigerator. This is when it compares to blood in terms of PH.

As a matter of fact, some of the potent foods that have anti-inflammatory properties and immune boosting properties, also work to empower the body to work to maintain its activities, including maintaining its ideal blood PH. I don't think this is a coincidence. Worth mentioning, it gets even more interesting, as some of these foods that empower the body, such as lemons, for example, are in their natural state, very acidic. However, their resulting post digestion effect after absorption into the body helps the blood to keep up with its slightly alkaline state. On the other hand, processed foods seem to work to affect this range toward a more acidic post absorption result, with the body needing to work harder through its various systems, to maintain its ideal PH.

Biologically, this system of maintaining an ideal PH, which the body typically does via complex processes through various systems, is empowered by what we eat. A diet, rich in fruits and vegetables (generally alkaline-favoring post absorption), has been linked with empowering the body to keep up with the maintenance of its ideal PH. Note that our proteins, although typically acid-forming post absorption, are also essential to our bodies because of the various other benefits they provide. This is so with certain other foods, as pertaining to the benefits they bring.

The *concept of moderation* can be applied in the use of *"tactful" moderation*, when dealing with obtaining the right benefits from our foods. I cited the two opposite effects to substantiate the fact that like the hot and cold-water scenarios, the mix ratios produce the overall effect. Generally, it's important to consider letting our ratios tip in favor of a relatively higher consumption of the alkaline-favoring foods for better immune health-boosting outcomes. In our application of *moderation* then, we can aim at *"tactfully"* taking actions that would favor an increase in our preferred side of the ratio. Note that in the literal sense, these foods do not directly regulate the blood's PH because of some of the complex processes I briefly mentioned previously, that are in place to do this fine work. However, the foods enhance and empower these processes. You can strategically consume the right foods to influence the process positively to your benefit.

Proven results cannot be denied, as you will see from some of the few food examples I discuss, and research studies that have linked benefits of certain foods to health. I choose to discuss these plant foods particularly because of their amazing health benefits to the immune system, and how easy they are to have available in your kitchen. I have included most of them on my list of favorite kitchen must-haves.

There may be several proposed hypotheses on how these work, but the basic thing to take away is, you are the result of what you eat. Additionally, my emphasis on describing the desired slightly alkaline levels of the blood PH is to help you to make some mental connection to this slightly alkaline desire even of our blood, as in relating to the choices of food we make. It's important to aim daily at making a relatively high number of food choices that favor an alkaline post absorption effect within the body.

Generally speaking, high amounts of consumption of fruits and vegetables as well as other plant foods, can be a great pathway to achieving this goal. Furthermore, remember that the end results of breaking down most foods prior to absorption are typically acidic. Examples, fatty acids from fats and oils, and amino acids from proteins are acidic. Additionally, the gastric acid produced in the stomach during digestion, which mixes with the food to aid the breaking down process, further stimulates an acidic environment. So, you see that acids play a role as well in the digestive process. However, the creation of an alkaline-favoring condition post absorption from the consumption of most plant foods make them desirable. This is because the overall result is important, and it greatly impacts the body's state of health.

As a quick tip, remember, that the processed foods and sugars will generally have an acidic post absorption effect, of which we generally have enough of. The foods with alkaline post absorption effect will help immensely to create good mixes (buffers) to give you the desired slightly alkaline effect; make choices that favor a high inclusion of those in your meals.

What is very beneficial for me, is to keep healthy foods as 85% or more of my general intake, whether daily or weekly. You can consider doing that as well. A general tip, at least a ratio of *85:15 healthy versus unhealthy minimum* daily or weekly (with tilts favoring the healthy side when necessary) is helpful to the body. Letting tilts favor healthy in the ratio whenever needed is a good one to keep in mind. There's always room for that 10-15% whether it's for a treat or an occasional sweet deal. And guess what, you get to choose how to use it, whether it's over a weekend, or spreading in bits a few times across your week. In your practice of this concept, you can start from wherever you may be right now, whether it's currently a 50:50, or lower. Make your current estimates, and work on adjusting ratios with tilts in favor of the healthy side. You can reevaluate your estimates weekly, and make necessary adjustments until you comfortably get into the ratio of 85:15 *healthy versus unhealthy minimum* or better. Don't be discouraged when you experience a few setbacks in the process. Just keep your eyes on your goal and keep pressing toward it.

Personally, I practice this by saving "junk" or "treat" consumption for family fun times, or gatherings with friends. These tend to happen on weekends or occasional weekdays. For that reason, I choose to strategically plan for those moments, saving my quotas for those times. For the most part, I try to stuff my refrigerator and home with healthy foods so I can be sure to keep up with my 85-90% healthy deals. Of course, I do have treats occasionally on those days if I choose to, but I keep them in moderation, with the whole picture of my week in mind, always leaving room to accommodate another need of junk consumption, should it arise during my week. I practice the *concept of moderation* via this tactic.

Additionally, there are also those times when I know the right thing to do is to say no, and I do. Even more so, when I know it's not healthy and I don't enjoy it anyway. Keep in mind that the tongue can be trained to dislike certain unhealthy foods, the same way it is trained to like them. This requires a simple choice to abstain for a consistent number of days, as you would with habits. Experts in breaking bad habits say a 21-day routine would do the trick, but with foods, I can tell you that many have seen success in as little as a week, as in breaking the habit of excessive sugar consumption. All it takes is the courage to decide, and the perseverance to pursue change in the right direction!

The key is having, or acquiring, a mental ability to stay in control of what you choose to eat or not to eat. This keeps the reverse from happening, as in the food being in control of you. There are many resources out there that help you to choose the right foods, and the right quantities as well. One of my favorites for general tips, that I usually recommend to my clients, is from Choosemyplate.gov.[1] This site from The United States Department of Agriculture has awesome general tips that can help you get up to speed with general everyday food selections. Be sure to check it out.

Do you remember the analogy of the chlorine added to the water in the swimming pool that makes available molecular substances which can kill bad bugs or germs? Another important aspect of creating the right environment in your blood is increasing the health-beneficial substances/molecules in your bloodstream that make it difficult for pathogens or even tumors to thrive.

Do you remember your basic little experiments in grade school and how substance dissolution in water affected the condition of the water's environment whether it was some sugar particles or even chemicals? Similarly, certain components from what we eat find their way into our bloodstream after their absorption from our digestive system. This can positively or negatively impact the condition of our bloodstream, depending on our choices. No wonder one of the major routes for making medication available in our bloodstream is via oral consumption. That is how powerful the digestive system is! As a result, even though the blood PH may not be directly and simply regulated by the alkalinity or acidity of what we eat, certain foods can further empower the body systems' ability to be effective with the process of regulation.

The foods we eat may have health-beneficial components or molecules, that can make their way into our bloodstream and boost our health. Therefore, it's not okay to simply eat just anything, every day. What you eat matters and can make a significant impact on the state of your health, as components break down and make their way into your bloodstream. To further explain this, let me use a scenario of when you have the doctor generally give you an oral antibiotic, for let's say, an infection. It's because components from this medication will get absorbed through the digestive system and make its way into the bloodstream, allowing it to "fight" the pathogens causing the infection. Bear in mind that the concentration of the medication consumed also matters, as the concentration that would be made available in the bloodstream also has a direct relationship with the concentration that would be orally consumed. This relationship is true, given all other factors which affect the absorption of that medication are properly in place. Together with other mechanisms of the body, the infection would resolve from the work of the medication that makes its way into the bloodstream. When the medication successfully completes its job, the infection is resolved.

Comparatively then, can you relate to the fact that the health-beneficial components from the foods we eat also go through this same digestive system and can become available in our bloodstream with necessary absorption factors in place? It's important to ensure efficient digestion and absorption of the foods we eat, so higher quantities of nutritionally beneficial components would be available in our bloodstream. For example, iron is highly absorbed in a Vitamin C-rich environment. On the other hand, calcium is, in a Vitamin D-rich environment. Hence, having the right nutritionally rich foods paired correctly in addition to many other factors can be very helpful in making nutrients available in beneficial quantities in our bloodstream. Foods that facilitate digestion and absorption of key nutrients when necessary and appropriate, can be potentially helpful to this process. That's why acquiring knowledge about foods is essential and can very well help with making the right decisions as to what to eat at any given time to attain maximum health benefits from what you eat. Chapter 25 throws a little more light that will help with this aspect of foods.

The foods you eat can boost your health or negatively impact it, depending on what your most frequent choices are. Remember also from the medication example, how much the concentrations matter to the medication's effectiveness in the bloodstream and body as a whole. In that same regard, what you put most frequently in your body can lead to an increased amount of its effect in your body whether good or bad. Your choices matter in determining the state of your health.

It is evident you can choose to use the everyday foods you consume to create an environment in your bloodstream where diseases would find it difficult to thrive. Some examples of foods that can help you achieve this effect are discussed as we go along. Keep in mind that there is a vast array of them. Take a moment to read a little more about some. This will help to increase your knowledge about them so you can get creative about using them more frequently to boost your health.

Some of what I discuss, I personally call basic kitchen essentials that can help boost your health. These foods, mostly plant foods, can be used to "spice" up your meals and health. I choose to discuss a few that are very common and full of amazing benefits. Always remember that there are tons out there, and these are simply what I call my definite must-haves, as they are very common and easy to obtain, although many times very easily overlooked. I share them with you so you can also consider obtaining them for your benefit. There is much more to explore.

CHAPTER NINE

Think Physical Activity

Obtain the benefits of a scheduled exercise
regimen by creatively incorporating other
beneficial options of physical activity in
ways that easily fit into your schedule.

My little steps count! Yes, they do! I know the first thing that pops into your mind when you see physical activity is scheduled exercise. Yes, it's part of it, but the concept of physical activity goes beyond the idea of performing a scheduled activity, as you will soon find out. For many people, the idea of exercise suggests a set of readily-scheduled activities, performed for one hour, and in the gym. This is wonderful, as many times seeing other people persevere through exercise motivates every one of us to do better. Going to the gym is great, and if you can, be sure to go regularly.

Usually, at certain stages or in certain seasons of life, when the demands on our time are not so pressing, it tends to be much easier to make time for scheduled exercise, especially planning for, and making a trip to the gym. As a busy working mother with an equally busy working husband, school-age children, and of course the demands of social commitments competing for my time, sometimes being able to make time to drive to a gym 20 minutes away from home even twice a week can be a real struggle. Trying to manage personal demands on time with regards to family, work, social and other aspects of my life tend to require great skill and balance.

Juggling your own schedules alongside those of your family and loved ones can demand a chunk of your time in a day and can be challenging in terms of even finding time to meet certain demands. However, this is an essential component of life that we must learn to accommodate. For many of us, the scheduled times for the gym is the first to begin to suffer a decrease, when we need to make room for other schedules as our responsibilities increase. As parents, we would rather take our kids for scheduled games than go to the gym if it means choosing one. That is a natural parental instinct and choice, and we should never have to feel guilty for making such choices. To complicate things, many of us find that we are exhausted by the end of the day, whether physically or mentally, from work and many other demands on our routine schedules. During these moments, the last place we want to be is at the gym on the treadmill, or on just any exercise machine. Typically, we simply want to do nothing in this state besides flipping channels to watch the news, which many times can also serve to increase the mental stress we may already be experiencing from our day.

For many people, this lifestyle can continue all week. However, it can get even more complicated from the guilt and discouragement of an inability to have been at the gym, may be as planned. Many people give up and correlate their inability to go to the gym as scheduled to an inability to exercise. Many more end up totally giving up on exercising once their scheduled plans to go to the gym are disrupted. Now, that is where the danger begins to creep in. Do you regularly think about the fact that your loved ones would love you to stay healthy for the longest possible time so you can continue to help them also make it to their next levels? For all the sacrifice and effort you are currently putting into making their lives better, whether it's working to pay the bills, or making time to visit with them to help them with their activities, they need you for the long haul. For this reason, taking care of yourself is very essential, and would benefit them also.

Think physical activity! That can help you to stay creative and obtain the benefits of exercise without the thoughts of a foiled plan to the gym when that happens. For example, planning for and engaging in mutually beneficial forms of physical activity as a family, as in taking walks, bike riding, jogging, etc. can be helpful and rewarding to everyone. You can creatively obtain the benefits of scheduled exercise regimen by incorporating other beneficial options of physical activity in ways that easily fit into your schedule. This is where physical activity becomes extremely useful, most especially on days when you cannot make the gym trips.

Physical activity can simply be any bodily movements that use energy in the process. In our homes, this could mean going up and down the stairs, mowing the lawn, playing, and running around with our kids in the backyard, swimming, walking, or jogging in the neighborhood, and many of the other options that may be coming to mind right now.

The *concept of staying physically active* can allow you to tailor physical activity to levels you can tolerate and/or incorporate into your daily schedules. Yes, this would encompass all forms of exercise as well, but staying mentally on this concept can help to make it easier, more fun, and doable for you. You can obtain physical activity by simply opting to walk up the stairs at work for even 5 minutes instead of using the elevator. The concept of focusing on physical activity helps and is personally very helpful to me. It stirs me into a mode of creativity and keeps me motivated in staying active as much as I can throughout my day, while also achieving great benefits as I would from scheduled exercises. Focusing on this concept can be very helpful, as it is one that can be purposefully thought of throughout your day.

Keep in mind that typically, physical activity can be vigorous or moderate. The Centers for Disease Control and Prevention (CDC) recommend adults get a minimum of 150 minutes of moderate aerobic activity, or 75 minutes of vigorous aerobic activity, or combinations of these weekly.[1] Generally, as a simple guideline, with moderate levels of activity, you tend to breathe deeper and harder than you would when you are doing nothing. At moderate levels of physical activity, you should be able to talk, although not able to sing consistently through a song without pausing to take a breath. You will usually experience some sweating a few minutes into moderate activity, as in taking a brisk walk in your neighborhood or mowing the lawn.

At vigorous levels of physical activity, your heart will usually be working at its maximum capacity, and your breathing would get even deeper and harder than you would at moderate levels. You will find it difficult to talk or sing. You would typically not even want to try to sing or talk, as you'll need to pause about every fraction of a second to catch some breath. At vigorous levels of physical activity, you break into sweating much quicker than you would at moderate levels. Activities at vigorous levels can include jogging in your neighborhood, biking, or hiking in hilly areas. As a caution, it's always helpful to start physical activity slowly if you've not been physically active for a long time. It's also very important to consult with your healthcare provider if you have any activity restrictions, as in the case of people with certain heart conditions. Your healthcare provider will help you to determine levels of physical activity that are safe for you.

Engaging in various methods of physical activity has many outstanding benefits to the body in addition to strengthening the body's muscles. To give an example as pertaining to the health of the heart (cardiovascular system), think about straws or even a water hose, which I compare to the arteries of the heart. Remember that as the blood flows through these heart arteries, there can be occasional accumulations of fatty components such as cholesterol in the linings of these arterial walls for many different reasons, some of which have been mentioned earlier, as in the consumption of foods high in "bad fats". This can lead to plaque formation and cause many potential health problems. For now, think about how these accumulations over a length of time can increase and gradually cause a narrowing of the diameters of these arteries. Eventually, this can interfere with the smooth flow of blood through these arteries and potentially block blood from effectively reaching various cells, tissues, and organs of the body. In certain instances, these arteries could narrow to an extent of totally inhibiting smooth blood flow to certain organs of the body. An inhibition of smooth blood flow to the heart can cause a heart attack.

When we exercise, like the water hose, we increase the pressure of blood flow through these arteries. This pressure many times can interfere with the formation of these plaques, as in the pressure from the water clearing little debris that may be along the walls of the water hose, or even straw as we suck liquids through them. If consistently adhered to, this analogy brings out only one simple possible mechanism by which physical activity can help to improve the health of your heart.

Physical activity can provide a wide array of "aerobic" exercises if we stay creative. "Aerobic" is very important to me in making an illustration here. Aerobic in meaningful terms has to do with oxygenation, and as pertaining to this discussion, making oxygen available to the body's tissues. Now, this is where I tie being physically active into building your immune health: *oxygen, oxygen, oxygen, let physical activity help its transport to your tissues.* Oxygen is very important to the function of the body, as it helps body cells to produce energy effectively. Simply think about how it fuels fires to burn more and connect it to how it can help your body to have higher energy. You could eat all the right foods, and ignore giving your body sufficient oxygen, and it will not be in good shape to produce the highest forms of energy.

Without going into the details about energy production in the cells of the body, I would try to put this in a way you'll remember. Simply, oxygen acts as fuel to energy production in your body. Next time when you've provided your body with all the right foods you can think about and are still feeling exhausted, consider exercising and see the difference that makes in how you feel.

My love for biology always brings me back to making connections from the cellular sense, and this time, using concepts from microbiology. The fact is, typically, a great majority of bacteria, viruses, and fungi cannot survive, or thrive, in an oxygen-rich environment. These do better in the absence of oxygen and are termed anaerobic organisms. This may be a needful idea to recall at this time, as I elaborate on the importance of oxygen to the body. Thus, boosting a good supply of oxygen to your tissues can help boost your immune system by simply creating an environment that makes it difficult for lots of harmful pathogens belonging to this group (anaerobes) to thrive.

There are certain advances in therapy which are currently utilizing an understanding of the role of oxygen in immune health enhancement, to help in certain treatments, inclusive of autoimmune diseases. A good example is in the use of the HBOT (Hyperbaric oxygen therapy). The HBOT is one that is heavily under research and has lots of studies that have shown it to be effective for treating autoimmune diseases in certain people.[2] In the use of HBOT in medical treatments, the body's ability to heal itself is heightened through a process, where individuals undergoing the therapy are given 100% oxygen within a total body chamber, while atmospheric pressure is increased and controlled.[3] HBOT is typically used in conjunction with other treatments that individuals who opt for may be undergoing.

Studies have shown that varying levels of oxygen plays a crucial role in influencing the degree of severity of the inflammatory response process, and eventually how effective an anti-inflammatory medication would be in mediating or stopping the process.[4] Relatively higher levels of oxygen have shown more positive results in comparison to lower levels. The use of the HBOT helps to further show how the body can even respond better to certain medications if individuals are able to do what is physically required to take those little steps that help with better oxygen availability to their cells.

I say all these to let you know you can boost your body's ability to heal itself or stay in good health, by boosting your immune health through the vehicle of physical activity. In my professional experience as a nurse, I can tell you that one of the major things that we tend to focus on, even for a patient recovering from surgery, is to help them go for levels of physical activity that they are able to tolerate, with any restrictions in mind depending on what their conditions or diagnoses are. We encourage even the littlest activity level when possible. There are so many benefits of this that it should not be overlooked.

All cells and tissues in the body benefit from physical activity; from the gut, right through every tissue, including tissues of the brain.

Physical activity, in addition to many other benefits, makes oxygen readily available to your tissues and boosts your immune health. Again, I continue to stress on the term physical activity because every little step counts. As helpful as the gym can be, you do not have to only wait to be at the gym to obtain benefits from physical activity. Personally, I have found that setting 10-minute goals interspersed throughout my day in engaging in physical activity helps me to do better at it. Whether it's during a lunch break or a deliberate time of play with my kids, it adds up. I have found that to be more doable and easier integrating into my schedule, and it also helps me not to feel guilty when I'm unable to carve out chunks of time on a busy day for exercise. I feel reassured even on those days that my 5- and 10-minutes count toward my optimal health goals for exercising at the end of those days. Consider this trick, and you'll be amazed at how much you're able to achieve.

Physical activity stimulates a release of the "feel-good hormones", endorphins (see Chapter 7), among the many other benefits to your health as in those discussed. Thus, your mental health and your emotions can reap benefits from physical activity. Mentally, people with anxiety disorders have seen improvement in symptoms from exercising.[5] A release of endorphins makes a huge difference in our mental state of health. Thus, we see that there are amazing benefits of physical activity to our bodies, not only physiologically, but mentally as well.

I remember during the season when I went through the challenge with my health, that at the time when I was physically able to get out of bed, taking little walks around the house, no matter how short or long those walks were, made me feel better mentally and emotionally. I highly recommend you do what it takes to stay physically active, even if it's for little amounts of time each day. Every little bit is better than doing nothing. Pause and think about some of the little things you can do during your day to get moving. Now, go ahead and formulate a plan that will help you to put those to work in boosting your immune health. Your body will thank you.

CHAPTER TEN

Rest To Gain

Foster creation and "recreation" of periods
of mental rest throughout your day.

W hy are you talking about rest when you just explained the importance of being physically active?
Yes, rest! I bet this time, from all the previous discussions, you realize that the ***concept of balance*** seems to be essential to immune health, whether it's in the foods we eat, or the
activities we choose to embark on. When I mention rest, I know
it's simple to think sleep. Yes, sleep is a major part of rest, and
very important. However, in this discussion, rest goes beyond
that. There are many definitions of rest, however, when I talk
about rest, I mean it in the context of "freedom from activity or
labor".[1] Rest can be physical or mental. This is where sleep can
typically take care of both, and the reason why sleep is invaluable to good health.

Getting adequate nightly rest via sleep is necessary, as this
helps our bodies to recoup from the "wear and tear" from daily

activities, giving it the necessary break to restore, replenish and reposition itself for subsequent activities the following day. Both quantity and quality of sleep are important.[2] It is essential to get adequate sleep at night, with the average hours totaling between 8-9.25 hours for most teens and adults. The National Heart, Lung and Blood Institute has an average recommendation of 7-8 hrs. daily for adults. 9-10 hrs. of sleep is recommended for teens, at least 10 daily for school-aged children, 11-12 for preschool-aged children, and 16-18 hours daily for newborns.[3] Keep these recommendations in mind, and work with your loved ones and family to ensure that your average sleep needs are being met. This will go a long way to help even the younger members of your family to stay attentive, focused, and productive in performing their regular daily activities, whether it's at school or riding their bicycle in the neighborhood.

I have come to realize that some days it's not easy to meet the daily minimum requirements due to heavier schedule demands. However, I have found it most helpful looking at my week's overall schedule and making sure that at least three out of the five weekdays whenever possible, I get as close as possible to getting the recommended nightly hours of sleep. I also find this helpful, especially for my school-aged kids. On other days, I try to help them not to veer too far off from the recommended guidelines when at all possible. Like most homes, we're not perfect at this but we aim for the best and use these concepts as a guide for making headway in the right direction.

Understanding why we ought to get enough rest is necessary for every one of us, young and old alike. Generally, toddlers and children have higher average requirements, with younger age groups having higher requirements as shown by the recommended guidelines. This is because a lot of body functions occur during those quiet moments, which help the body to maintain itself in a healthy state. These functions include the release of growth and appetite-regulating hormones, muscle repair, memory strengthening functions[4], and much more. These necessary functions require an uninterrupted period of nightly sleep, based on everyone's unique needs.

Let me use some analogies to paint the necessary picture of what happens with inadequate rest. Have you ever cut back extremely on the number of hours you sleep at night? Now picture what happens to you during the daytime, following those nights. It is usually difficult to concentrate and get the mind to perform at its maximum, whether it's in performing work-related activities, or even activities necessary for meeting some of the most basic needs in extreme situations. There is a lack of energy necessary to keep you engaged mentally and physically in performing activities at your usual maximum capacity. This is mainly because all the steps necessary to complete the major functions related to restoration, replenishment, and repositioning the body for our next day's activities are not completed when we lose hours of sleep. This leaves the body short of being ready for maximum performance the following day. For children, especially babies and toddlers, inadequate sleep can even affect their growth, as this is a major function that is active during sleep, whether it's got to do with brain cell growth or the growth of other body parts.

It's no wonder we tend to see even the skin respond negatively with signs of early wrinkling when adults experience prolonged periods of sleep deprivation. You enhance the beauty of your skin with adequate rest. Of equally important significance to me is the fact that a lack of adequate sleep has a detrimental effect on your immune health, with the opposite being true.

Studies have shown that prolonged interruption of sleep stirs an initiation of inflammatory processes in the body referred to as chronic low-grade inflammation, which also negatively affects the immune system and the body's overall health.[5] As a matter of fact, there are certain components of the immune system's function that are active during sleep as well, as in the action of certain T-Cells. In addition to the other roles they play in the body, these T-Cells have a major part in acting to boost the body's protective function. We can tell this easily, as the body is generally better able to fight infections, even as seemingly slight as the common cold, when given adequate rest. Adequate sleep is an essential component of the body's rest regimen, and it's important to give your body the number of needed hours of uninterrupted rest it needs especially nightly. This will help to boost your immune health and enhance your overall health.

As much as adequate sleep helps us get most of the rest our body needs to keep up with daily demands, it is also very important for us to keep in mind the importance of mental rest even while we are awake. Taking advantage of your body's ability to increase the secretion of "feel good hormones" (endorphins) can go a long way in creating an internal mental environment of rest. There are many activities that can boost their production. Carefully review Chapter 7, where these "feel good hormones" are discussed, and consider using them to your advantage in boosting your immune health and the overall health of your body. Foster the creation and "recreation" of periods of mental rest throughout your day as you review this chapter.

Empower Your Brain To Rest

Many times, when you hear about eating healthy, the first thing that comes to mind for most people is getting rid of fat from our diet. Let me mention that this is only partially right. You know by now that the key is "balance". For instance, while trying to keep your cholesterol levels in check, what has been found to be one of the most effective strategies has to do with not only getting rid of saturated fats from the diet (which tend to increase Low-density lipoproteins, known as LDLs or "bad cholesterol"), but replacing them with foods that are high in monounsaturated fats (which tend to raise your High-density lipoproteins, known as HDL(s) or "good cholesterol").

Generally, most sources of saturated fats are those from animal fats as in the fats from our meats, dairy products, butter, etc. This is a major reason why I strongly recommend you eat lean portions of meat, trimming, and discarding visible fats. Furthermore, consider taking off and discarding the skin from your poultry whenever possible, before consumption and/or cooking.

These general tips can help immensely in decreasing the amounts of saturated fats you consume. Be sure to pay attention to food labels when available, to see content for these different types of fat. Decreasing fats in your diet should be true for saturated fats, as they tend to cause the issues when they make their way into the body. A low consumption of saturated fats is essential to decreasing "bad fat" levels in the body.

There are also the trans fats, which are also a component of what I'd term the "bad fats". When you think of these trans fats, think about the major source being from partially hydrogenated oils used for deep frying most foods in fast food restaurants, as well as those used in most baked pastries, doughs, snacks, and those found in margarine, etc. The high amounts of trans fat content is a major reason why these foods should be consumed minimally. Trans fats may also be present in certain quantities in foods that are rich in saturated fats. Saturated fats and trans fats together form the major components of what I call, the "bad fats". We should be mindful of consuming these in very minimal quantities. I always say that we will have the minimum requirements of those in various forms made available in the body, even when we try to keep our consumption of them low.

Obtaining the beneficial nutrients from milk, or our meats that come along with trivial amounts of fat after we've put in place all the necessary checks to trim our meats or drinking our milk with say 2% fat versus whole, would still introduce those low amounts of "bad fats" in our diet anyway. Therefore, we need to take measures in other instances, as in being careful to eat foods that are generally low in these "bad fats" to maintain our overall consumption in very low quantities. A helpful tip would be to fill up on healthy meals before proceeding to grab a small piece of dessert like cake on a day when we crave for it, and not making such occurrences every day, at every meal. There are many more you can come up with, just by getting creative.

Your brain needs "good fats" consumed in small to moderate amounts, to stay in good shape. It is very important to be attentive to consuming moderate fats from foods rich in monounsaturated and polyunsaturated fats. These are mainly fats from plant oils, like those from seeds, nuts, avocados, as well as oils from fish oils such as salmon, mackerel, sardines, and much more. These mono and polyunsaturated fats are sources of "good fats". Monounsaturated fats are generally liquid at room temperature and begin to turn solid when chilled. Examples are fats from avocados, peanuts, olive oil, etc. These are the most preferred. Polyunsaturated fats, on the other hand, are liquid both at room temperature and when refrigerated. They are typically contained in sunflower, and certain oils obtained from many nuts and seeds as well. What is also very notable about these "good fats" is that, in addition to helping nourish the health of your brain, they also boost the function of many other organs and systems in the body, such as the heart. As you can see, they are worth paying attention to, most especially when the amounts of "good fats" your body needs are comparatively small but go a long way in enhancing the performance of key organs and systems.

Small to moderate consumption of "good fats" coupled with moderate amounts of protein and foods rich in fiber will keep your tummy feeling full for longer periods. This is because digestion of these foods is not as quick as in that which occurs when you eat processed foods and empty calorie-dense foods. These unhealthy "junk" foods will also get you to crave more for them, creating a cycle where your tummy would always want frequent refills, because of their quick digestion and the lesser creation of fullness in the stomach. Keep in mind they are typically filled with loads of "empty" calories. These are quick fuels for weight gain and health problems. Fortunately, you can train your body not to crave for them even if you find yourself in this cycle. All you need to do is fill up the healthy way consistently for about 3 weeks, and you'll notice a difference you'd be glad to perpetuate.

This is a wonderful tip for healthy weight management. Be sure to pay attention whenever you eat your major meals of the day whether it is breakfast, lunch, or dinner. Being attentive to fill up right, helps to decrease the need and quest for frequent unhealthy snacks. Whenever you must snack, throw in a few fruits, vegetables, and nuts, and you will notice the difference this makes in helping you eat healthy, delicious foods, while also maintaining control over what you eat, and not the other way around.

"Good fats" provide key nutrients that play a major role in the development, growth, and maintenance of the brain and nervous systems. In pregnant women, during periods when major growth advancement is projected with the brain and nervous systems of the developing baby, a corresponding increase in consumption of fats, preferably good fats, is recommended to the mother to be. I state this to help further bring out the importance of consuming foods rich in "good fats", and the impact it has on the health of the brain and other systems of the body, even at the level of development of a baby in the womb.

You can find very good information and resources that can help you make good choices when it comes to fats and general heart healthy nutrition from American Heart Association.[6, 7] Explore options at your leisure from their website. My aim is to provide a broad understanding so as to make the little details easy to deal with in your everyday encounters and choices. With this broad understanding and tips at hand, I believe making choices pertaining to the consumption of fats in your diet when you are faced with them will be much easier.

Keep in mind that healthy brain cells will do what they must do when the occasion demands them to perform. Whether it's in helping you keep up with your memory or other cognitive functions, or simply producing hormones that will help you to feel good, giving your brain good nourishment is vital to helping it stay in good shape and performing necessary functions. When the brain is nourished to stay in good health, its proper function can help to boost your immune health.

When you eat fats, opt for sources of good fats, and your brain, immune system, and your body at large will thank you. When your brain is well nourished, it is also able to perform the functions necessary to empower the body to rest. Whether it's in sleep function, or stimulating a mental state of rest, or even performing any other body functions that would feed into boosting your immune health, it lies within your means to feed your brain with the right nutrients, including "good fats", to help it do what it does best. This will help to ensure that your brain continues to function at a maximum capacity, most especially when you need it most.

CHAPTER ELEVEN

The "Boss Of Your Body"

Having a mindset of being "boss of your body" gives you confidence to have what you want at the time you want it, and on your own terms that are right for you.

It's very important for you to have plans in place that will help you discipline your body well enough to be able to incorporate healthy choices into your lifestyle. This understanding can be even more helpful to you when it's based on knowledge of what you can put into your body that can foster a boost of its immune health, whether it's got to do with food or activity. You are the steward of your body, and who can take better care of it than yourself?

The concept of being "boss of your body" is one I practice purposefully. I would highly recommend for you to have this concept somewhere at the back of your mind when it comes to making daily choices. We all have feelings and cravings that sometimes try to get in the way of us wanting to make the choices we know can boost our immune health. Many times, we fall for making frequent choices that do not support the health of our immune systems instead of the other way around. How many times have you decided to eat ice cream more frequently than you know is best for you? If you're not an ice cream fan, think about a dessert choice you love to make frequently that is not necessarily the healthiest for your body, and picture that.

Now, how many times have you decided to eat this dessert and have gone overboard, eating more than you would have liked to, and then fallen into a feeling of guilt? Do you identify with any of these situations? Feelings of guilt that result from making such uncontrolled decisions, have a strong tendency of lingering in your mind even long after you've acted upon these decisions. For many of us, they have a potential of getting us distracted as we focus on them so much, instead of thoughts we could have obtained from eating these foods controllably. It deprives us of the potential enjoyment and satisfaction we could have obtained from having eaten such foods. This can contribute to a negative feeling and mood, instead of a desired positive feeling and mood.

How about this one: how many times have you felt strongly about eating something that's unhealthy but at the same time felt like it's not the right time for that "treat" but have simply overlooked your thoughts and gone after your feelings and felt guilty after that?

You must be getting what I'm trying to portray by now, that there is a clear difference between your feelings and the rational thoughts that originate from your mind. Many times, these two very much oppose each other. However, practicing the use of the *concept of being "boss of your body"* can help you to personally take control of both your thoughts and your feelings, while purposefully maintaining control over who "runs the show" in your body. Personally, I love to always think about the fact that God created me in His image to be in control of what He has blessed me with. I can do all things through Christ who strengthens me.[1] With that in mind, I also know that I can gain wisdom from His word to take care of my body, which is His temple and of which I am a steward.[2] As a good steward, it's very important for me to take charge and take good care of what I have in my care, and in this context, my body. Gaining knowledge and understanding is essential to everyone's ability to be the "boss" of their own body. You are making time to read this book, and this is a good indication that you are taking the right steps in the proper direction.

I can tell you that to be successful at being in control of your body, you must be mindful of any conflicts present at any given time between your rational thought processes and your feelings. Many times, our feelings can get in the way when it comes to the need for making healthy choices. An approach I've found personally helpful in handling this issue, is first acknowledging the existence of any such conflicts in these different domains, when confronted with options to make healthy choices. For example, I may have an idea to go for a walk to get some exercise on a day when I feel exhausted, and also just want to sleep. At that time, my feelings may be in the way of me taking that walk, although I know rationally that doing this would help enhance my mood and set me on a better track for good sleep later. Acknowledging the existence of such conflict within me would help me better move forward, instead of ignoring this conflict and simply allowing things to go in just any direction. Do not deny or dismiss the existence of such conflicts, or they will hide in your subconscious mind and present themselves as a challenge whenever you're faced with making similar decisions in the future. Acknowledging the existence of these conflicts can help you to deal with them based on the knowledge you've acquired. This can also help you to put to rest any "irrational" feelings that do not need to prevail, or even thoughts in certain circumstances that do not align with the right knowledge you've acquired. The right knowledge you've acquired can either align with your existing feeling or with your rational thought. Know that it can go either way. This can leave you with a stronger thought or feeling based on whichever wins in terms of being in alignment with the right knowledge you've acquired.

The winning side, whether rational thoughts or feelings, will end up staying dominant in your mind. Let's assume thoughts win for this scenario, as usually, the conflict exists in a stronger sense when the feelings are not in alignment with what you know to be true. Many times, rational thoughts would tend to infer from the knowledge you've acquired, whether right or wrong. There are still many other times when your "gut" feelings/thoughts set in to reinforce the strength of your regular rational thoughts. These "gut" feelings tend to be those that you know sometimes are right somewhat but are not able to pinpoint the reasons for them being right.

In dealing with "gut" feelings, you should realize that you can sometimes engage with them, especially when your rational thoughts do not totally align with the right knowledge you've acquired. For example, you want to eat two large scoops of ice cream when you simply feel that eating this would bring satisfaction to you but are neglecting any health-related consequences you know of. At this time, you realize your "irrational" feelings have been set into motion, and you need to be mindful of an existing conflict. Mentally, you may recognize your rational thoughts in action, arguing that the sugar content is too high, and may not add much nutritional value to boosting your immune health. This argument may stem from you remembering what you know about your immune health and high levels of processed sugar.

You may recall that high levels of sugar can fuel the inflammation processes in your body, and you may be swayed toward doing otherwise. You may decide that it would be better for you to eat some fruit to fill up and eat a scoop or less of the ice cream later, or not at all this time. You realize your rational thought process wins this time. Your "gut" feelings may simply say to you, "don't do this", without much to back what it's indicating but that of "it just doesn't feel right". Based on the right knowledge you've acquired about eating too much ice cream and its potential effect on your health, both your rational thoughts and your "gut" feelings will end up not aligning with those "irrational" feelings, but you need to allow your rational thoughts and "gut" feelings to win.

When your rational thoughts and "gut" feelings are continually trained to win they make the most sense. They are then happy to come back to defeat any "irrational" feelings when the occasion arises again. With a few repetitions of this process, your mind becomes stronger, you get to "be the boss" and your "irrational" feelings are no longer allowed by your body, to rule. Very soon, you'll be amazed at how these "irrational" feelings will not be as loud when they kick in, because they do not receive as much attention from you as they did before. With time, they will no longer pose as much of a strong challenge to your "healthy" decision-making processes.

On the other hand, you can dismiss this conflict between your thoughts and feelings and let them linger until you suddenly find yourself eating the huge bowl of ice cream without giving much thought to it. It's important to think about your thoughts and feelings, especially if they appear to be in conflict with each other. You see, in such decision-making processes, all it takes to start practicing this concept is a one-time ability to become conscious of acknowledging the existence of a conflict between your rational thoughts and your "irrational" feelings.

Using the base of the right knowledge you've previously acquired about the subject of the decision you need to make, as from the outlined example, you'll be able to make a healthy, winning choice. Repeating this process a few times over and over will lead to the use of this concept becoming a part of your decision-making processes. This will help you keep the title of "the boss of your body".

There is an important concept that ties in closely in the effective use of the major concept of being the "boss of your body". I term this the *concept of gratification-at-will.* I use this sometimes, and I find it helpful in maintaining control over "irrational" feelings and thoughts as pertaining to food choices. I subtly demonstrated the use of this concept in the two huge scoops of ice cream example. This concept can be used to rationally take charge and "negotiate" with your "irrational" feelings, the terms you'd prefer to go by. In fact, most times, you'd need to "dictate" the terms of your preference to your "irrational" feelings, and not "negotiate".

For example, your decision to eat some fruit to fill up and eat a scoop (or less) of ice cream later would be a great way to feel a 'better you'. The next step after "dictating" better terms with your "irrational" feelings in the use of this concept, is making plans that would have a potential of decreasing or even "neutralizing" some of the potential consequences of this seemingly negative decision. In this example, you can commit to not eating sweets the rest of the week or cutting back on your regular amounts in quantities that would make up for what you are eating at the time. Use of these two concepts (the *concept of gratification-at-will;* and *the concept of being "boss of your body")* hand in hand, will then bring you back on track to what your normal sugar intake regimen should be. In arriving at good "dictating" terms in this example, you can use ideas from our discussion of the concept of using the *minimum of 85:15 "healthy versus unhealthy" foods ratio* with your daily or weekly (whichever you choose to use) intake in mind (see Chapter 8).

Keep this in mind as you make meal plans over the week or month, to stay mindful of not consuming excessive sugar by other means or being very reasonable and conservative with consumption. The use of these concepts allows you to handle your "irrational" feelings reasonably while also maintaining control. This can be very helpful to you when it comes to staying the "boss" of your body. This strategy allows you to stay in charge satisfactorily, versus allowing your "irrational" feelings and thoughts to lead you overboard.

Having a mindset of being the boss of your body is very helpful, knowing you can confidently have what you want at the time you want it, and on your own terms that are right for you. The use of this strategy also helps to gain an afterthought of having met your need and laying it to rest for a period. This can leave you with a happy feeling and a potential ability to secrete feel-good hormones, which can help boost your health. This is completely opposite the guilt that could result from following the dictates of your "irrational" feelings alongside the consequences from the actual choice.

Portions of food consumed at any given time do matter to the health of the body. It's important to be mindful of that and stay in control of the portions you eat. Of course, occasionally, you may eat a little above your normal portions, as during certain family occasions or celebrations. However, it's important to make those truly once in a long while, and not a daily practice. Also, when you choose to eat these foods, make sure it's truly your decision to do that, and you are not being swayed by your "irrational" feelings. Stay the boss!

CHAPTER TWELVE

Spice Up Your Health

*Your immune health, no matter its current state,
can be spiced up into better performance.*

It's amazing how much impact your kitchen can have on your health, depending on how you choose to use it and what you fill your kitchen with. There are amazing simple natural spices and herbs that can enhance and support your body's immune health. You can obtain great tasting foods from many of these, while empowering your "defense hub" to do what it has been wired to do.

I found out that cleaning our pantries, getting rid of spices with chemicals, and simply replacing those with our very basic herbs and natural seasonings, can go a long way to promote our health. There are many "seasonings" on the market these days that are sold to help us have better-tasting foods, tenderize our meats, or simply do anything we want to with our foods, to enable us cook faster, and so much more, for our convenience.

Among many out there, monosodium glutamate (MSG) is a very popular and controversial one that has been a subject of debate for many years. This is one that is a component of many processed foods as in certain chips, and lots of commercially sold seasonings for the kitchen, aimed at enhancing the taste of our foods. MSG has been linked to headaches and certain allergies.

There are lots of research studies that have highlighted its potential impact on health. A popular one featured by the International Journal of Clinical and Experimental Medicine carried out by Xiong, Branigan, and Li, highlight findings that led them to a conclusion that MSG's headache-causing potential "may be related to its effect on brain neurons".[1] Their findings also led them to conclude that low doses of Vitamin C intake can potentially prevent, or decrease some of MSG's side effects. I mention this research work because it goes a long way to enhance my previous discussion of the fact that putting in place measures that boost your immune system can help your body to better mount a defense mechanism against "intruders", such as an exposure to potentially harmful chemicals, as in this example. More so, discussions in Chapter 3 highlight Vitamin C as a powerful immune health booster, among others.

There are many ways we are exposed to chemicals and toxins on an everyday base. From the air we breathe, to some of the foods we eat, to even the after effects of regular exercises that we don't have much control over. Toxins can be introduced subtly into the body by various means, whether from active or passive activities we carry out daily.

Did I really mention exercise? Yes, exercise! Many of your body's functions would naturally release toxins, including muscle stretches from exercise. The body would rid these toxins in various other biological functions as from those you would experience from sweat and much more. As with previous discussions, there are many good things we do, or things we introduce into our bodies from certain foods, that have unwanted by-products that also rely on what we do or put into our bodies as from foods, to enhance the body's ability to get rid of them. The body is naturally wired to perform many of these functions, and we can boost its performance by arming it with good nutrients from the foods we eat. I mentioned exercise, very important to our health, to bring out the fact that many times, we do not have control over the modes of exposure to certain toxins, as sometimes some of this exposure can be a by-product from some of the good things we do for our bodies, such as exercising, eating, driving, swimming, and much more.

Your body is wired to naturally rid many of these toxins, if it is well-armed to do so. The Centers for Disease Control and Prevention (2009) Fourth National Report in Human Exposure to Environmental Chemicals, outlines a testing of 212 chemicals, an increase of 75 chemicals from its previous edition.[2] This to me indicates a possible or actual increase in chemical exposures to humans, as well as a corresponding elevation in the awareness of a heightened exposure for a higher number of chemicals, in comparison to tests performed in its previous edition.

I believe that our aim should be to do our best to minimize our bodies' exposure to chemicals, while at the same time increasing our body's ability to defend itself and stay healthy despite chemical exposures that we do not have control over. As simple as it sounds, our kitchens, from the hearts of our homes can help us to do both!

Take a moment. Look at that spice rack sitting on your kitchen counter, or anywhere else you've placed it in your kitchen. Do you know what spices are on there? How many times have you used or even thought of using any specific one(s)? Do you have any favorites? Now look around in your refrigerator and anywhere else you normally store your fresh spices. How often do you use these? Do you have any favorites in particular? If I tell you that some of these could help boost your immune health, would you believe it? Now, although there are many, I am going to make a few picks in the next few chapters, elaborate on those, and I hope this will stir you up to begin to explore plant foods.

Some of them are my favorite basics, and I hope you'll consider making your personal picks from these and much more out there. Yes, your immune health, no matter its current state, can be spiced up into better performance. When your immune health is spiced up, your health as a whole, benefits from it. In addition to the various concepts discussed, the practice of food-related concepts can be enhanced, using examples from certain simple foods present in the average kitchen that have immune health-boosting capabilities. These will help you to put some of these concepts into quick practice. Many of these foods are often easily overlooked and underutilized.

CHAPTER THIRTEEN

Ginger

Simplify processes, stay efficient and effective in managing your health

Ginger is one of my favorite natural spices, and I use it very often in my kitchen. Its scientific name is *Zingiber Officinale*. This amazing plant is one that flowers and tends to grow over a period of about 8 to 10 months. It grows predominantly in tropical climates, although conditions can be created anywhere to grow ginger. In the U.S.A, a lot of ginger is grown in Hawaii, as the climate favors its cultivation. We generally consume the rhizome, which is the part of the stem of the plant that grows horizontally beneath the surface of the soil.

In the grocery store, ginger is typically displayed close to other root vegetables such as turnips, beets, etc. Likewise, it's important to clean ginger very well and peel them like we would other root vegetables. When shopping for ginger, I look for one that's as smooth as I can possibly find, as it makes it easier and quicker for me during the peeling process. Additionally, the ones that feel firmer are typically fresher. The weightier it is, the more flavor there is from it. In shopping for ginger, I look closely and select the ones that are best-looking, the same way I'll do with other fresh vegetables, inspecting for potentially rotten spots, and avoiding those.

Why Ginger?

In addition to the robust unique flavor and taste that ginger brings to many dishes, especially when freshly cut up or blended in food recipes, ginger has long been known as a potent anti-inflammatory and antioxidant. Among others, gingerol, is a popular bioactive substance that affords ginger its "medicinal" properties. Scientific studies support the presence of gingerol and other bioactive substances in ginger.[1] Having such amazing health benefits, it's no wonder that many people have reported its great benefit to their digestive health. I have personally experienced many benefits from ginger as well, inclusive of the benefit of aiding digestion.

Ginger has great popularity as possessing anticarcinogenic properties, with various research studies supporting that. Anticarcinogens are substances that have an ability to negate the effects of carcinogens. Carcinogens are substances that can cause cancer in living tissue. On the flip side, anticarcinogens are generally also referred to as substances with potential cancer preventive capabilities. Ginger's active ingredients like gingerols, shogaols, and paradols, are great substances that can prevent various forms of cancer.[2] Studies have shown pancreatic cancer cell growth to have been inhibited, both inside and outside of experimental animals used in studies, by the activity of the medicinal constituents of 6-gingerol and 6-shogaol.[3, 4]

Digestive health can benefit from ginger. Gingerols have been proven to provide the antioxidant properties of ginger.[5] Yes, there is so much research study that supports ginger's medicinal capabilities! Gingerol has been shown to have an ability to hinder the invasion of certain breast cancer cells, a major type of human liver cancer cells (known as hepatocarcinoma cells), as well as other cancer cells, demonstrating a capacity to cling to these cells in the process (showing motility and adhesion properties).[6,7]

Ginger is an asset to your digestive health. I have personally heard many people report relief from nausea; it helps even some pregnant women with morning sickness. In fact, it has been successfully used in a study as an antiemetic (a substance with prevents vomiting), in preventing nausea and vomiting during pregnancy and chemotherapy in certain people.[8] Others have reported obtaining soothes from upset stomachs, and I can attest of this, as it is one of my major useful quick fixes for indigestion, both for myself and for my entire family.

Ginger's anti-inflammatory properties have been beautifully shown through the pain-relieving effects it has proven in certain studies. Findings have shown that women with painful menstruation (dysmenorrhea) can find pain relief both in intensity and length of time, from ginger.[9] It can decrease muscle pain following intense exercising.[10] Ginger can improve cardiovascular disorders[11], diabetes mellitus[12, 13] and gastrointestinal health.[14]

It's benefit to the gastrointestinal system is easily seen even in seemingly trivial situations as in relief from flatulence, indigestion, and much more. From lots of supporting research studies with only a few cited to help communicate its value and potential benefits, we see that ginger has great health-enhancing benefits. I believe it's a spice that should always have a strong presence at the heart of our homes. My idea of many disease processes and how they start at the cellular level, particularly those that have got to do with the inflammation process, help me to put in proper perspective, the need to consume more foods with anti-inflammatory properties. Doing this I believe can better arm the body to fight the start of many disease processes, thus, boosting the immune health. I can tell you that ginger is an asset to me and it can be to you also.

A tip for exercise lovers like myself who also sometimes dread the general muscle soreness that comes along with exercising, especially after taking a long break from it, is that ginger can be a helpful escape for you! Ginger and extracts from its family, such as curcumin from turmeric have been shown to delay exercise-related pain from muscle soreness.[15] Again, its anti-inflammatory properties in action.

Ginger has demonstrated strong effective anti-bacterial activity in some studies, in combination with other natural spices with similar properties such as garlic, cloves, etc., against some multiple drug-resistant clinical "bugs" (pathogens).[16, 17] A lot of studies, with only a few cited, have seen some of the most potent antibacterial activity of ginger in combination with other natural spices. I always think of the idea of "eating the rainbow" as pertaining to eating our fruits and vegetables, with the most benefits obtained when more varieties of colors are consumed. In the same manner, I believe we get amazing benefits from eating a wide variety of health-beneficial spices from the heart of our homes.

In some places of the world, I believe that some people do not experience certain diseases when they eat and drink contaminated foods and water, just because of the combinations of spices they consume from some of these range of potent spices with antibacterial activity. A study from Bangladesh supports this.[18]

In the winter, there are many like myself and my family who obtain great health benefit in staying on top of cold-related respiratory infections, simply by keeping ginger close to the heart of our home. Warm herbal teas or fresh juices with spoonfuls of my favorite paste made with ginger are my preferred drinks during the winter season. I believe they do a lot for me in strengthening my immune system and minimizing my chances of getting severely under the weather, especially while in constant interaction with people who have frequent coughs and colds. Even when I happen to come under the weather, this awesome mixture helps to shorten the length of time, so I can keep up with the pace of daily demands during the winter weathers.

Initially, I shied away from ginger because I was not sure of how to effectively use it, store it, as well as how to consume a decent amount to obtain its benefits. I know many identify with this as well. As a lover of plants, I began to quickly learn to shop effectively for ginger, just after I learned about its great benefits, and the tips I described earlier have been of great help to me in buying ginger. As soon as I began to use ginger, I realized that no amount is too small not to use, whenever I have the opportunity to do so. I simply place my ginger from the grocery store in a resealable ziplock bag, making sure it's dry. Sometimes, I even leave them in the clear plastic vegetable bags from the grocery store. I always make sure the ginger is thoroughly dry, so it doesn't begin to go bad quickly, as I tend to store them for long periods with an aim of making sure I always have some in my refrigerator.

For any cut portions, I make sure I blot those dry. Sometimes, I poke little holes in the bag if it's a large quantity. I anticipate condensation and moisture accumulation during the initial periods of refrigeration in the vegetable drawers, and the holes usually help to minimize this potential dampness. I recheck after about 24 hours when they are cooled to the desired temperature. If there is an accumulation of moisture, I blot them dry and change the storage bags. Again, my goal in all of this is to ensure the absence of moisture so it would last longer during storage. I also make sure to get rid of as much air from the bag as possible, as this also helps to keep it fresh for longer periods. I've kept fresh ginger in my refrigerator safely and good-looking for up to about 6 weeks, with good refrigerator temperatures in my vegetable drawers.

I always love to simplify processes, to help me stay efficient and effective in many ways, given the many demands on my time. I know it's the same for many of us. In spite of the many competing strains on our time, it's important to go the extra mile and do what is necessary to keep up with taking care of our greatest God-given assets, our bodies. Now, I keep a few on the go mixes refrigerated most weeks, so I don't have to blend ginger daily, especially on busy weekday nights, should I need some for myself or my family. This is especially useful to me in the winter months. My favorite recipe is making what I call my "Ginger-Apple Paste":

Ginger- Apple Paste

I add a tablespoonful or more of this Ginger-Apple Paste to water, sometimes apple juice, or any juice of my choice, or a warm mix of water and honey. Occasionally, I add this to some of my favorite herbal teas in hot drinks as well, especially during the winter seasons. Other times, I eat the blended mixture by itself, depending on my preference that day. My family does the same, and we explore many options each day. I hope you and your loved ones can do the same also.

Ingredients:

- Peeled, sliced ginger: ¼ to ½ cup

- 1 Medium-Large Apple of your choice

- 1-2 tablespoons of freshly squeezed lemon juice

Preparation:

- Wash your apple: I love to do this by first rubbing vinegar on the apples for about 5 minutes and then rinsing them (great way to prepare your apples before eating them); or pouring boiling hot water over them when placed in the sink or in a bowl, to help wash off most of the wax coating and potential pesticides. Then I rinse them with plain tap water. You can try any of these options.

- Next, core your apple by removing the seeds and cutting them in sizes ready for the blender.

- Place your cut-up apples and ginger slices in a blender

- Add about an ounce of water to make it easy on the blender. You can add a little more water depending on the quantity of your blend and your preferred thickness.

- Add your lemon juice and simply blend to your preference of smoothness. I like to get it as smooth as possible, as this makes easier for mixing with drinks. You can substitute the water with your favorite juice that mixes well with apple and ginger. You can't go wrong with using apple juice.

- Pour mixture into an airtight container and store in the refrigerator, using 1 or more tablespoons as per your preference, with your drink mixtures.

Taste and Preferences:

- The number of ginger scoops to use will depend on your preference and the amount of spiciness you can handle, as well as the quantity of the mix you would want to add to your drinks for any single serving. Generally, the more concentrated the ginger you have in your paste, the less you may need to fetch in your drink preparations, to get to the tolerable level of spiciness you can handle. Thus, feel free to adjust to suit your taste and preferences.

- Usually, a medium sized rhizome gets me about a 1/4 cup when sliced. My mixtures tend to last me about 7-10 days if taken continuously in small quantities of about 1-2 tablespoonfuls when adding to my drinks.

- The lemon juice is simply to help decrease the rate at which the mixture begins to change coloration (oxidation), as you'd normally see in a cut-up apple over a certain period of time. Hence, the lemon juice helps the mixture to last longer without quickly changing color. If you prefer an extra zesty flavor, you can add more lemon juice during preparation, or at the time when you are ready to add to your choice of drink. Lemons are full of great health benefits, and sometimes I add some more, especially during the winter, on days when I feel under the weather. Again, adjust to your preferences. Enjoy!

CHAPTER FOURTEEN

Turmeric

Find innovative ways whenever possible,
to facilitate absorption of targeted foods
for greater potential health benefits.

Turmeric belongs to the ginger family, *Zingiberaceae*. I call it a cousin of ginger, because of its origin, and the closeness of its benefits to that of ginger. They are usually next to ginger in the produce section of the grocery store. Shopping for them and general refrigeration for storage, for me, tends to follow the same patterns as for ginger.

It is a valuable spice found in many spice mixes like curry powder. It looks just like ginger on the outside but what differentiates it from ginger is its additional yellow coloration. This yellow coloration is produced by naturally occurring phenols in turmeric, popularly known as curcumin. Several other components have been isolated from turmeric, a major one, turmerone, which is a volatile oil.[1]

The beautiful yellow coloration of turmeric is used by many in the food industry to obtain food coloring benefits. Food products like curry powder, mustard, and relish, to name a few, tend to benefit from this yellow coloration. It is no wonder it has great popularity in many regions around the world. Its prevalence in curry powder makes it a popular spice component in many cuisines around the world. There are many great recipes with turmeric out there, as well as for ginger.

However, despite its great healthful benefits, many people, including myself, tend not to be able to consume it in large quantities at any single time due to its sharply strong, somewhat bitter taste, unlike ginger. I tend to do supplements whenever I need more turmeric, always exercising a lot of discretion with quality in selecting those as in the purchase of any other nutritional supplements. This is an option that should be used discretionally. Make sure to consult with your physician, as in the use of any other food supplements.

Why Turmeric?

The use of turmeric's health benefits in a medicinal fashion dates back over four thousand years.[2] As in ginger, turmeric has been known to possess outstanding anti-inflammatory properties and has long been used popularly in Chinese and Ayurvedic medicine. Turmeric also has great antioxidant properties, which is also reflected in its great benefits to our health.

Outlining a few of the numerous health benefits of turmeric will help to really show the value it can bring to our health, right from the heart of our homes, our kitchen! As a nurse with many years of experience working with patients, including those who have undergone surgery, I understand the importance of pain-relieving agents and the significance they have on the healing process, especially when taken with an aim of minimizing potential side effects. Many of the potential side effects from our traditional pain-killers tend to continually pose a challenge in their use, especially if they are used for long-term pain management. Of course, do not overlook the fact that high doses of some plant remedies could potentially interact with the function of some of our regular medications.

I love to always err on the side of caution and say that whenever in doubt, always check with your healthcare provider. Yes, even with supplements! I always tell the clients I coach to discuss the subject of pain relievers with their healthcare providers, especially if they have to undergo surgical procedures. One of the questions I always recommend them to consider asking when they talk to their healthcare providers is the effect of the pain medications they take, and whether they can supplement or gradually wean off to natural pain relievers if they choose any; to discuss specific choices, as well as any potential interactions with any medications they are taking, and any cautionary measures they need to put in place. This is very important, as from my clinical experience, I realize that patients who take proactive measures in managing their pain effectively, especially with plans in place, tend to have a better drive in performing other tasks necessary for quick recovery. These tasks can include walking and deep breathing exercises to aid recovery especially after a surgical procedure. It's amazing, but I can tell you that it's the little pieces of the puzzle that make a great impact on our overall health. Be proactive and pay attention to those little things!

Now, one of my favorite research findings with regards to the medicinal properties of turmeric has got to do with its pain reducing properties. In one study, patients who had undergone a laparoscopic cholecystectomy surgery were given high doses of curcumin (2000mg/day).[3] These patients obtained significant pain reduction within a period of 1 to 3 weeks, compared to patients who were not given the curcumin supplements. There goes the potent anti-inflammatory property on display! It's interesting to say that even low doses of turmeric intake (72mg and 144mg/day) have been found to significantly reduce abdominal pain associated with irritable bowel syndrome.[4]

Even the little amounts of turmeric we consume, whether in our foods or as supplements, can make a significant difference in the state of our health. The pain-relieving effect of turmeric extracts (in doses of 1500mg/day) has been shown to be as effective in treating pain in patients with knee osteoarthritis, as that of ibuprofen, 1200mg/day over a period of 4 weeks of monitoring these study-participating patients.[5] Turmeric is one of my valuable healthful spices from my kitchen. Many times, I use turmeric as my first line of support for minor headaches to minor body aches and pain, and I get great results.

Turmeric's anti-inflammatory property has been found to have a protective effect on the liver cells of patients receiving methotrexate for treatment of cancer.[6] Among other reasons, a lot of patients take methotrexate for Rheumatoid Arthritis because of its great benefit to them as determined by their healthcare provider. Some get concerned over time because of its side effects. A major side effect of methotrexate is its potential toxic impact on liver cells, which results in their careful administration and management by healthcare workers, especially at high doses. Thus, it's great that turmeric could help in alleviating such potential toxicity.

Studies have found that using different dosages have indicated the safety of curcumin as high as 12g/day over 3 months.[7] Curcumin has been proven to have beneficial properties that interfere with the growth, specifically the invasion and migration, of cancer cells.[8] Its limited toxicity and safety to humans in addition to its anti-cancer properties[9, 10] make it a valuable asset. This outstanding property makes it very beneficial to people willing to try natural avenues of boosting their health, especially when undergoing invasive treatments.

Keep in mind that discussing the possibility of using a wonderful natural supplement like this with your physician who has knowledge about them, most especially if taking any prescribed medications, is always helpful. Your physician may be able to consider some of these and further provide advice that could additionally potentiate healing benefits of any prescribed treatments or medications.

Since there are so many diseases that arise from the inflammation process, as this is typically one of the body's natural initial means of defending itself against diseases, it is not surprising that many well-documented health benefits have been discovered that can easily be traced to the anti-inflammatory properties of turmeric. People with stomach disorders usually associated with the inflammation process as in Inflammatory Bowel Disease (IBD), or Crohn's disease, or Ulcerative Colitis, may benefit from consumption of turmeric in their diet. Studies have shown that curcumin constituents positively affect a couple of gene variants linked to IBD's severity.[11] Additionally, curcumin extracts have shown muscle relaxing effects in the intestines of experimental animals studied.[12] This effect could well be an additional contributing factor in relieving IBD symptoms in people who have benefited from it.

Many more benefits of turmeric have been discovered. I have only highlighted a few major ones pertinent to some of the common concerns most of us tend to deal with on daily bases. There are many more pointers to the possibility of even more potential benefits of turmeric extracts and which lots of resources have not yet been dedicated to researching. The area of the study of the effect of curcumin on neurodegenerative diseases (such as Parkinson's and Alzheimer's) is one I believe if more resources are put into, could potentially make a noticeable difference for those who struggle with this disease. I say so because indicators have links to its favorability in alleviating some symptoms related to this group of diseases.[13]

A diet rich in curcumin or its derivatives has been shown to alleviate symptoms of Post-Traumatic Stress Disorder (PTSD).[14] Positive results have been shown in its use in alleviating depression.[15] Curcumin has been shown and said to potentially help in healthy aging of the cardiovascular system.[16] Again, I believe the antioxidant and anti-inflammatory properties play an active role in all these. Think about the fact that most of these neurodegenerative diseases occur because of the inflammatory process getting out of hand to begin to fight the body's healthy cells. There are some that even negatively affect brain cells sometimes in various ways. I have heard amazing testimonials of outstanding benefits many have obtained from including turmeric in their dietary regimen, whether in foods or as occasional supplements.

Curcumin has also shown great antimicrobial activities in studies, a very popular one of which is related to *Helicobacter pylori (H. Pylori)*, a type of bacteria that causes stomach conditions as in peptic ulcers and some other gut-related symptoms of infection.[17] It has also shown both some antiviral and antifungal activity with certain strains of flu virus and fungus. *Candida albicans*, a common fungus that causes yeast infection in women resulting in itching and burning sensation in the "female tract", has responded to turmeric's active fight. Many other viruses and fungi (in addition to the ones mentioned) have succumbed to the potent action of turmeric.[18, 19, 20] In my opinion, this spice is a must-have in our kitchens!

My take, trying the consumption of turmeric in inflamma-tory-related disorders can be beneficial to anyone and may be worth the try. And yes, the inflammation process can target any organ in the body and has been linked to many chronic illnesses to which curcumin has been shown to have therapeutic poten-tial benefits. These include diseases such as Alzheimer's disease, Parkinson's disease, multiple sclerosis, epilepsy, cerebral injury, cardiovascular diseases, cancer, allergy, asthma, bronchitis, coli-tis, rheumatoid arthritis, renal ischemia, psoriasis, diabetes, obe-sity, depression, fatigue, and even AIDS.[21]

As a healthcare worker, seeing so many people suffer from debilitating diseases usually chronic, and which also affect their quality of lives, I am passionate about increasing awareness of such assets in our homes. Many times, unassuming but poten-tially able to provide so much value to our overall health in boosting our immune health, some of these great plant foods have so many benefits we can take advantage of. My joy is in the fact that I believe God has made available to us a wide variety of these, so that perhaps, if one does not obtain benefit from one natural food, another could work for them if only they do not give up trying and searching for what works uniquely for them.

Carefully consider giving turmeric a place in your home. Like ginger, turmeric and its curcumin constituent have been placed by the USDA on their Generally Regarded as Safe (GRAS) list.[22] It's very popular in the food industry in coloring foods, from cheeses to mustard. So far, scientific studies have not demonstrated any toxic effects either in humans or animals from the use of turmeric.[23]

A major challenge has been in its minimal absorption in the gut when ingested orally, thus, decreasing the availability of cur-cumin and its related substances within the bloodstream. Many scientists discuss this in terms of the subject of bioavailability whenever this poses a challenge, when it comes to food and other substances of similar interest. My personal experience is that many foods aren't totally absorbed when we eat them together. For example, our iron would compete with calcium for absorption in the gut when foods containing them are eaten together. This is due to the "competing" and close relation of the charges of these elements in their chemical activity, a subject beyond the scope of this discussion.

Many of us can benefit from finding innovative ways whenever possible, to facilitate the absorption of targeted foods we consume, by creating an environment that makes the food's absorption rate higher within the gut. For me, an example of this could be in the consumption of my Vitamin C-rich foods or supplements, with my high iron-containing foods, or consuming calcium with Vitamin D, whenever possible. I try to be strategic, although eating all these together sometimes is no problem, as some nutrients will find their way by all means into the bloodstream. Of greater value however, get creative in enhancing benefits from absorption by being mindful of appropriately pairing complementary foods whenever possible.

We do take some medications with food just to have them bind to these foods and have the body absorb them better. My illustration of these absorption-related ideas is to say that I would not let the absorption challenges within the gut deter me from consuming turmeric, as this is not new to many of the foods we eat, and even some of the medications we consume. The body will find a way to absorb some, as exemplified by the many studies where oral consumption of turmeric has proven beneficial.

I get creative, as in taking with meals when in supplemental forms, to have my body mimic its absorption as though it was in actual food. And yes, I get great benefits from it, and I believe anyone can also obtain benefits from turmeric. Consider getting some turmeric. And be sure to read the bonus chapter on tips for "Mixing Right".

As a general tip for shoppers of turmeric supplements, in addition to exercising all the necessary quality checks, also look for the addition of black pepper. Black pepper has been shown to have a component, piperine (also branded as Bioperine), which aids the absorption of turmeric within the gut (also see Chapter 25). This is a step in the direction of progress, in helping with the absorption challenge I mentioned earlier. Turmeric is another great product to consider using to your advantage, from your kitchen!

CHAPTER FIFTEEN

Cayenne

Enjoy life: try not to make eating a burden, but one you enjoy and maintain control over.

C ayenne is a common spice in many kitchens, as it tends to incorporate this zesty taste and "feel" to dishes. Like most of us, I tend to purchase this spice from my local grocery store from the spice aisle, and it usually comes in powder form. This is one of the most common states as it stores very well on spice racks.

Cayenne is made from chili peppers, a member of the Capsicum family of vegetables. In this form, the chili peppers are typically dried and ground to a smooth perfection. They are the same that come as the crushed peppers which we usually use as additional seasoning either during cooking or after cooking to get an extra taste of "spiciness" as we typically say. I also buy cayenne in the crushed form. There are still times when I buy the fresh chili peppers and make them into a paste form, blended together with other spices of my choice such as onions, and incorporate into various recipes of my preference during cooking. This paste form is also carried in our local grocery stores mostly in the aisle that carries spices for Asian dishes. When I buy this form, I read labels carefully, trying to keep preservatives and other unhealthy additives to a minimum. When I buy the fresh chili peppers, I usually keep them in freezer-safe Ziploc bags and store them in the freezer, sometimes for over a period of 2-3 months, using them in crushed, paste, or smoothly blended forms in some of my favorite recipes.

When I think of cayenne, I simply think of "spicy" peppers. I like to use various kinds of spicy peppers, and I tend to try a wide range, as there are so many of them: Habaneros, scotch bonnets, jalapenos, just to mention a few. I use them in various recipes, from jalapenos in my salsas, to habaneros in various stews. I simply try them, as they tend to add variations to the flavor and taste of my foods and make them taste different and great.

If you are as daring as I am, keep trying them by simply substituting the various peppers in your recipes that call for spicy peppers. Believe me, you'll find various varieties you like, while also enjoying the health benefits they bring to you. This is what I do; at the grocery store, I look out for people buying peppers or other vegetables I like to try. I ask them for their personal favorite recipes. When I come home, I find various variations of these recipes whether from cooking channels or cookbooks, that suit my preferences. Involving your family can be a great way to explore new recipes. They can enhance your ideas and help tailor those to the family's preferences. I love to involve my family in such "adventures", and I'm always amazed at some of the great new recipes we are able to come up with. This can help not only in exploring healthy homemade recipes, but also enhancing good family eating habits, most especially in the younger members of the family who are picky eaters. This can go a long way in helping instill in your family, an ability to stay open to trying out new and healthy recipes if that is your focus like mine. This will stay and last with them a lifetime.

For the scope of this book, I focus only on cayenne peppers as pertaining to peppers, but I encourage you to try a variety, a few of which I mentioned earlier, and obtain the many benefits they can bring to your health. Keep in mind the fact that some may not be spicy, as in our bell peppers and many others including the grilling variety. These can also bring good benefits to our health, as displayed by their various beautiful colors. Explore and enjoy them!

Why Cayenne Peppers?

Chili peppers used to make cayenne, contain bioactive nutrients known as capsaicinoids. These nutrients have been attributed to great weight management boosting capabilities in certain individuals, as it specifically aids in increasing energy expenditure, increasing lipid oxidation, and reducing appetite.[1]

I have reviewed various research studies on cayenne and they have affirmed my opinion that cayenne is great in supporting weight management and should be used to the extent tolerable in diets. Individuals who are actively using diet, exercise, and other proven methods of weight management to further boost their weight management effort can obtain great benefits from this spice if used in right and appropriate food quantities.

Imagine going to your favorite pizza restaurant with a friend and ordering your food. Now, both you and your friend decide to sprinkle some crushed peppers on your slices to the extent you're able to handle the spiciness. My question for you: Do you think you'll both be able to handle the same amount of spiciness? Let me take it a step further to create this same picture for spicy wing lovers. To what extent are you able to tolerate the spiciness of hot wings as compared to a friend or a family member? I can compare the degree of cayenne's heat to that in spicy wings because spicy peppers are used to formulate varying degrees of the heat index in the wings preparation industry. I am driving home the fact that this great spice should be used in careful adjustment to individual needs, as different people can tolerate different levels of spiciness.

Some people go an extra length to take cayenne pepper in capsule form, especially for some who realize great results in relation to weight management. I would personally not take cayenne in pill forms or recommend that anyone should do that because of the absence of the effect of spiciness on the tongue of individuals who would take it, among many other factors. This can interfere with the possibility of regulating to accommodate tolerable amounts of pepper in various individuals. However, as a useful helpful tip, the frequency of cayenne consumption is key, which has been linked to a decrease in abdominal adipose tissue levels.[2] This could be a result of cayenne's help in burning fat. I like to simply put tolerable amounts in my foods, and that is helpful. I always love to paint the total picture so everyone has useful information that would help them in making great decisions, especially in relation to their health.

In 2012, there was an isolated incidence of a 25-year-old young man being presented to the Emergency Room with severe chest pain after using over the counter cayenne pills in his attempt to lose weight. He was diagnosed with an acute heart attack (myocardial infarction).[3] With other factors ruled out, cayenne pills were attributed to be cause. The cayenne pills could have caused this young man's heart condition because of a component of cayenne pepper, capsaicin, which has an ability to stimulate the components of the body, responsible for activating the "fight or flight" response (the sympathetic nervous system).

I believe the stimulation of the "fight or flight" response was at a much-increased level in this young man, although it's also a way that cayenne works to bring about its positive effects.[4] This was documented as the first incident linking the use of cayenne pepper pills for slimming, to the cause of an acute heart condition.

I cited this isolated incident because of my personal preference of eating cayenne in endurable amounts in foods regularly, in order to obtain benefits, as opposed to taking it in pill form, although I totally understand that some individuals realize benefits from that. I usually encourage the former among my loved ones, friends, and clients I coach or talk to, when this subject arises. Additionally, everyone is unique, and has a body system that may respond in different ways than another person's when presented with the same exposure, and can be true, even for foods. My personal thoughts on life and its relation to food are simple: Enjoy life, and try not to make eating a burden, but one you enjoy and maintain control over.

Some of the notable benefits of the components of chili peppers, including its capsaicinoid components, are found in its medicinal (pharmacological and physiological) properties, which include the activities of pain-relieving effects (analgesia), anti-cancer, anti-inflammation, antioxidant, and anti-obesity.[5] Therefore, capsa-icinoids contained in chili peppers may be potentially beneficial in the area of pain relief, cancer prevention, and weight loss.[6] As a matter of fact, capsaicin, another biologically active compound in red chili, can slow the growth of cancer cells, suppress the inflammatory response, and may likely be a key mediator in cell death or destruction (apoptosis) pathways, in certain human cancers.[7]

Because of such great benefits, I enjoy keeping this spice in my kitchen. It will be worth giving chili peppers a chance in your kitchen too, especially if you enjoy spicy foods. Enjoy the benefits it can bring to your health. As mentioned earlier, it will be helpful in limiting this wonderful spice to your dietary intake and watching out for levels of what your body can tolerate while at it. By all means, add some heat to your favorite recipes, the way you like it.

CHAPTER SIXTEEN

Lemons

Make deliberate attempts to teach children
good habits including those from eating. This
will help them in forming healthy personal
opinions that will last them a lifetime.

L emons are fruit from the species *Citrus limon*, which
belong to the Citrus group of plants like oranges and
tangerines, to name a few. These fruits tend to grow
their best under warm temperatures and full sunny conditions,
making them popular in tropical and subtropical humid regions
of the world. In the U.S.A., California and Florida are the most
popular citrus-growing regions.

I love lemons and I'm always very excited when I get to talk
about them. I call lemons one of my kitchen's must-haves. Like
many others, I love the taste of lemons, and my kitchen does
not run out of juices from lemons. They come in handy, from
using them to boost certain seasonings in some of my favorite recipes, to occasionally adding them to my water and other

drinks to enhance their taste. Many of my fish recipes taste even better when I add lemon juice to them. There are tons of recipes out there that make use of this amazing fruit. Adding the juices of lemons occasionally to some of my smoothies typically result in various great tastes as well that keep me wanting more.

It's important to remember that like many citrus fruits, lemons may not mix very well with certain foods, as in milk. Be sure to keep this fact in mind, especially as you try different combinations of fruit and vegetable smoothies, with an option of including lemons every now and then. There are tons of smoothie recipes also in many cookbooks, on food channels, and online food networks. Be sure to explore the many that utilize lemons and find ones you enjoy most. When it comes to foods, you will certainly find your preferred combinations. Make sure they are ones you enjoy.

I have various ways of storing lemons. I typically get them fresh from the fruit aisle in my local grocery store. I put them dry in resealable Ziploc bags and keep them in the fruit tray of my refrigerator. Some have lasted for me, as long as a month. Some are able to last for a few days simply in my fruit basket on my kitchen countertop. Some people prefer to store them in this manner and buy them in relatively fewer quantities.

When freshly squeezed, and refrigerated, I can keep lemon juice for up to about a week. As a busy mom with a need to also keep up with demands of work while also keeping up with the health of my family, getting freshly squeezed bottled lemon juice sometimes from my local grocery store is also always a plus. I make sure to check the ingredients to ensure the juice is pure with no additives and stick to getting organic brands, as this helps me to feel safer about a decreased possibility of having pesticide contaminants introduced into the juice, especially during the squeezing process. You may find that the bottled form also comes in very handy. It does for me, as I use lemons very often. There is always a way to make lemon juice available in your home, in ways that suit your personal preferences and needs.

Why Lemons?

Lemons are a rich source of Vitamin C, a primary water-soluble vitamin that also acts as a great antioxidant in our bodies, as discussed earlier. Remember, antioxidants can act as "scavengers" of free radicals (see Chapter 3). Like many of its citrus fruit "counterparts", lemons can be a good source of some amount of dietary fiber and does contain a rich source of flavonoids (compounds in plants that are of benefit to health) such as naringenin, hesperetin, and many others, just to name a few. These flavonoids empower the body to fight diseases. Lemons also have traces of various other health-beneficial nutrients, as in vitamins and minerals like Vitamin A, potassium, zinc, etc.

Lemons are one of the kitchen essentials I find helpful, which can aid the body in its maintenance of, what I discussed earlier, the slightly alkaline PH in the "Swimming Pool" (refer to Chapter 8). This slightly alkaline PH I believe, is conducive to creating an environment that makes it difficult for germs and other disease conditions that can initiate in the body, to successfully perpetuate themselves (also see discussion in Chapter 8). And yes, sometimes undesired, and unwanted conditions in the body could be in the form of a tumor that begins to form, someplace in the body.

Lemons are naturally acidic in nature. However, after consumption and absorption of its components into the body, lemon is able to provide an environmental state that tilts toward favoring an alkaline state within the body, where it's able to provide amazing health benefits. In fact, raw extracts from various parts of the lemon plant (leaves, stem, root, flower) have been shown to possess anti-cancer properties and antibacterial properties against clinically relevant strains of bacteria.[1,2]

Let me throw in the fact that most of your citrus fruits, such as your basic oranges and tangerines, originating from the same citrus group from which your lemons belong, have been demonstrated to have amazing health benefits. These citrus fruits, and which scientists classify in certain instances together as Citrus limonoids, and which include lemons of course, limes, grapefruits, oranges, pomelos, mandarins, and bergamots, have been studied and shown to demonstrate lots of medicinal properties, some of which are anti-cancer, antidiabetic, antioxidant (of significance), antimicrobial, insecticidal and much more.[3,4,5]

A way to remember the connection between the antimicrobial properties of lemons and their citrus counterparts, and their ability to potentially benefit the body in this regard, is in this demonstration: Many at-home cleaning supplies tend to have lemons included in their ingredients, taking advantage of their potent antimicrobial properties. To add a further connection, can you think about any common cold remedies you know? Now, think about cough drops and lozenges. Have you noticed how often most cough drops and lozenges use the potent properties of lemons to potentiate their healing capabilities?

To add a few more, lemons are also great in helping with good weight management.[6,7] Obesity statistics are increasing rapidly within our societies, most especially in recent times. Such valuable foods should not be overlooked. There is also a concern about growing obesity among children and teen populations. Obesity has been shown to have a major link to many chronic diseases such as heart disease, diabetes, and much more. Helping and teaching children to include and fill up on healthy snacks is very important, most especially in this era. Adults would benefit immensely from this action also, but I mention this to emphasize on the importance of paying attention to our children, as they innocently tend to emulate habits they often see around them, whether good or bad. Make deliberate attempts to teach children good habits including those from eating. This will help them to form healthy personal opinions that will last them a lifetime. In turn, healthy personal opinions will influence them to make positive choices, no matter what they see around them. Guide your children and you'll be amazed at the difference this guidance will make.

Citrus fruits, such as oranges and tangerines, can provide significant amounts of fiber for the digestive system when eaten often. This can also contribute to increasing a feeling of fullness, and decreasing excessive food consumption, especially from those containing "empty" calories. In the end, it helps with better weight management. In addition to encouraging intake of citrus fruits by making them available in your kitchen, you can also help your family consume more limonoids and take advantage of their health benefits by finding creative ways of including them in recipes in your kitchen.

As caution, stay wary of excessive sugar consumption whenever using lemons in your drinks so you don't end up with higher sugar intake in an attempt to consume more lemons. This is because most drinks that use lemons as in lemonades, also tend to add lots of sugar to them. Beware, read labels, even if it says 100% juice, no sugars or preservatives added, or any other attractive wording on the label. I usually add lemons to plain water, and it tastes great. As a healthier alternative to sugars in lemonades, I generally add lemons to fresh 100% juices, and my kids love it as well. Consider giving this a try by adding to some of your favorite juices, and I believe you and your loved ones would enjoy that. And again, water is the best drink!

Drinking lots of water can help with avoiding excessive intake of calories from sugary beverages. This is also a very valuable tip when it comes to healthy long-term weight management. Many have had great benefits from drinking lemon in warm water first thing in the morning. I do that occasionally, and I sure love the vitality I obtain from lemons. Like any foods, be cautious of any allergies, especially when consuming for the first time. I realize that lemons help a lot with digestion, and it's amazing the relief I obtain when I feel like I have challenges with indigestion. It's even better when I take a spoonful of my mixture of ginger blend with the lemon juice in it. It does wonders for me. Consider giving this a try the next time you have challenges with indigestion before reaching for over-the-counter medications.

With kids in my home, I can't tell you enough how much my favorite ginger-apple paste blend with a hint of lemon (see Chapter 13) is always a blessing with occasional upset stomachs. Of course, and as usual, be cautious in ruling out any other possibilities other than just a minor stomach discomfort from indigestion before using the mix, or any at-home remedies in general. This is because some ailments can present themselves with such "murky" symptoms. Be sure to contact your healthcare provider if you determine a feeling of possible indigestion may be stemming from other causes, and more especially if you do not find relief from at home nutritional remedies like this.

Can you think of just how much of a difference this will bring to your health if you paid attention to making sure you have lemons and citrus fruits in your kitchen? Paying attention to consuming them, even if about a couple of times weekly, can enhance your immune health. What a difference this could make to your health if you simply tried to find recipes and also make substitutions in recipes to include some of these citrus fruits.

There are tons of quick healthy recipes you can make that include lemons. From guacamoles to smoothies, through fish seasonings and all the in-betweens. From drinks to sides, appetizers, and dinners, you can seamlessly find means of using lemons in your kitchen to enhance your health. And by all means, eat the oranges and other citruses to further boost the benefits of these lemons.

CHAPTER SEVENTEEN

Garlic

The little opportunities you take advantage of
can make a big difference in your health.

Garlic is a potent vegetable that grows underground in the form of a bulb. Scientifically, it is known as *Allium sativum*, belonging to the class of plants with a bulb-shaped formation, as in chives, onions, scallions, and leeks. Each bulb of garlic consists of cloves that are arranged in such a special and unique way that they come together to form the bulb.

When I think of garlic, I always think of onions because of the similarity of their bulbs, although onions do not have the singular partitions that form individual cloves like those found in garlic. The cloves can be easily pulled apart individually, as each is covered separately by a thin sheath. The number of cloves needed can be taken apart from the whole bulb for any single use.

Garlic and onions share a close relationship in origin, looks, and use. They have very popular culinary uses, because of the unique flavors they add to foods, and many times tag along with each other in certain recipes. From mashed potatoes and various types of bread, sides, and appetizers, to meats like chicken and much more, garlic and onions are able to add a robust flavor that can transform and change the outcome of a meal to something amazing. This is the reason many of us find it useful in classifying garlic as a spice in our kitchens.

Some people classify garlic as an herb, and I believe it's because of its medicinal value and uses. Sure enough, you can also choose your own method of classification based on the value it brings to your health and home. I personally agree with all these different use-based classifications. This is because I have varying uses for garlic as well, and at any given time, based on what I may be using it for, garlic would be in line with any of these classifications. In my kitchen, garlic is king, and I always make sure I have some in the house.

Garlic is prevalent in Central Asia, although it's grown all over the world, because of its superior culinary uses. In the United States, California is one of the nation's largest producers of garlic. Like many vegetables, fruits, and herbs, lots of people enjoy growing garlic from their own gardens and backyards. If you love to garden, this may be worth the try. Just be sure to get the right garlic cloves to grow from your favorite home and garden store. The grocery store-bought ones may have undergone processes that may not make them qualified candidates for planting; they may not sprout in most cases.

In the grocery store, fresh garlic can easily be found in the produce aisle, usually close to onions. Like many of our spices, garlic can also be found in dry forms in the spice aisle. Given that it can be used in various recipes both in the fresh form and in the dry form, I make sure to carry garlic in both forms in my kitchen. Like all of my spices, I carefully read labels to ensure I purchase high-quality forms of powdered garlic when I shop.

As in onions, when buying fresh garlic, it is very important to inspect the bulbs carefully to make sure they have no molds or softened spots on them. Feeling the bulbs for firmness is important as well, as I have realized that firmer bulbs of garlic are able to store longer, and those that feel soft or have a shrivel-like appearance tend not to last as long. Beware, and choose firm, good looking garlic bulbs. Fresh garlic can also be bought in minced form, bottled in jars, from the grocery store. These can then be kept in the refrigerator after opening. Whenever you need to buy garlic in this form, be sure to read labels, looking out for preservatives. Generally, those with minimal preservatives do not last as long, once opened and refrigerated. Keep that in mind when opting for this this alternate form, also being careful to read instructions on storage and how long you can keep after opening.

I can tell you that one of my most valued kitchen utensils is my garlic mincer. I spent quite a few bucks buying a good quality one because of the frequency of use, and I can say that it's been worth it. It affords me the opportunity to quickly get minced garlic, fresh, and on the go for my recipes when I need it. It also saves me time from lengthy periods of mincing and dicing. There are many quality garlic mincers out there on the market. Consider investing in one, and you'll be glad you did. It will come in handy when you go for recipes requiring minced and diced garlic. You'll be amazed at how efficient these good garlic mincers are, plus, you get your garlic fresh for these recipes, cooking tastier meals.

Storing garlic is one of the easiest to do, as it does best and stays longer when simply placed loosely in a basket at room temperature. The great thing is, if you buy the firm healthy-looking bulbs, they'll last the longest for you. Simply placing the bulbs in any basket that allows proper ventilation at room temperature, will help your garlic last even longer. I have successfully stored fresh garlic for up to a couple of weeks. Beware of conditions that could stimulate sprouting or mold formation in your garlic, typically moisture-generating conditions. This could include storage in an airtight plastic bag or container, or even refrigeration for long periods.

I have also obtained success in storing garlic bulbs for about a month, with these bulbs placed loosely in the vegetable drawer of my refrigerator. I believe fresher ones can go even longer. Most importantly, always remember to keep your garlic away from moisture-generating conditions. Additionally, I would recommend you stay away from freezing your garlic. I have discovered this is simply a bad idea. It becomes extremely soft when taken out of the freezer and does not add as much of its good flavor to foods as needed in that condition. It literally loses most if not all of its flavor, and I believe the value as well. For your dried garlic, storing is very easy. Simply place them wherever you place your dry spices, as on your spice rack or place of preference in your kitchen

Why Garlic?

Garlic has been used for many centuries as a home remedy for many ailments. There are documented uses of garlic as home remedies as far back as the 18th century in Europe.[1] From worms in children to fevers, bronchitis, and much more, folk medicine has experienced amazing health successes and benefits from the use of garlic as remedies.

To give you a simple good idea or mental picture of the outstanding medicinal properties of garlic, let me tell you as a lover of plants, that even some gardeners utilize its potent properties to ward off small pests like aphids, insect larvae, etc., from their "organic" gardens while trying to stay away from using toxic pesticides on these vegetable gardens. Some gardeners obtain success from this by making a mixture of crushed garlic and water, allowing this to soak for about 6 hours plus, and spraying it on their vegetable plants. The benefits are awesome, as garlic has a natural ability to repel insects. I describe this use, to illustrate the natural potency of garlic, and the remarkable benefits it can potentially bring to your health if you begin to deliberately incorporate it into your recipes.

Over time, life has become very modernized to the extent that many things have evolved to make it easier for us to keep up with the fast pace of our very busy lives. For this reason, it has become very easy for us to sometimes overlook the great benefits we can provide to our health from simply consuming some "simple basics" such as garlic, and the few others I have mentioned.

I am a firm believer of the fact that a return to the consumption of some of these basic foods can help to curb some of the trends in the rise of debilitating chronic diseases within our society today. You should not only work on informing yourself about all-natural remedies, but also empower your children (along with many generations down the road), to stay informed when it comes to the choices they make with their foods, and the impact it can have on their health.

Garlic's great health benefits stem from its bioactive components. Garlic has a peculiar smell and color that typically comes from allicin, a high sulfur-containing compound that is formed from certain sulfur precursor components of garlic, when it is crushed, minced, chopped, etc. Allicin has antibacterial and antifungal properties with demonstrated benefits to health. It is interesting to state that allicin does not occur naturally in garlic but its precursors are present. When garlic is processed as in mincing, crushing, chopping, etc., the precursor components are activated to produce allicin, which in turn produces the unique smell that adds flavor to our cooking.

There are other health-beneficial bioactive components of garlic that are worth mentioning outside of its sulfur-containing components. Among others, arginine and selenium are worth mentioning. Arginine, an amino acid that converts to nitric oxide, is a powerful neurotransmitter (chemical compounds that work to transmit impulses) in the body that aids in blood vessel relaxation and is known to improve circulation, even in heart arteries.

If you happen to know people who have been determined by their doctors to be at a high risk for heart attacks, you may know some of them to carry nitrate-containing medications on them. They usually place this common form of the medication (sublingual) under their tongue, when they experience chest pain. This is because of the relaxing effect nitrates can bring to blood vessels, making them invaluable to managing certain heart (cardiac) conditions. This analogy is helpful in aiding the formation of a mental picture of the potential benefit of garlic consumption to the health of the heart.

Selenium is an essential mineral typically found in the soil. It is also known to have great antioxidant properties that prevent cellular damage in the body. Selenium is known to play a great role in helping to boost the immune function of the body. Among others, it also helps with heart and thyroid health. Like many others, selenium can be found in a wide variety of foods such as chicken, eggs, beef liver, spinach, turkey, sardines, brazil nuts, and much more. This supports the earlier discussion that proposed the necessity of eating a wide variety of healthy foods and the benefit of this action to health. The presence of arginine and selenium in garlic is definitely worth mentioning.

High consumption of garlic, as well as others within the group of allium vegetables (such as onions, scallions, and chives) has been linked to a decrease in risk of certain forms of cancer. This is because of antitumor activities found in this group of vegetables. In recent studies of nutrition, dietary interventions and their relations to prostate cancer, a relationship between heart and prostate health has been discussed, with some therapists of prostate cancer patients generalizing "heart health equals prostate health".[2] Do you see here the importance of boosting your immune health and its potential positive effect on various other systems and organs in your body, including your heart?

A study conducted in China of patients diagnosed with prostate cancer supports the fact that a high consumption of allium vegetables such as garlic, onions, scallions, and others in the group can lead to a decreased risk of prostate cancer, with the most significant results being as high as a 50% decrease in risk, obtained from consumption of quantities greater than 10g per day.[3] Additionally, in this study, people who were at earlier stages of the disease benefited most, in comparison with those at the late stages. It is best to always consume lots of foods that boost your immune health as this could do so much in supporting your body's ability to fight disease (Chapter 8). This research study and many others mentioned, go a long way to support this concept.

There are various other forms of cancers whose risks have been shown to decrease with consumption of allium vegetables. Some studies have demonstrated that a high consumption of allium vegetables, especially garlic and onions, has a protective effect against stomach and esophageal cancers.[4, 5] A protective relation between raw garlic consumption and lung cancer has been shown to exist.[6] The antitumor activities of garlic have been shown to be effective against certain breast cancer cells.[7] Garlic and onions, particularly uncooked onion components, have the capacity to suppress multiplication of a wide range of cancer cells by decreasing the ability of the cell cycle to progress, and/or stimulating natural destruction of those cells.[8, 9, 10]

It is no wonder we see its potential to decrease risks of certain diseases, as in some forms of cancer, with extensive studies done and continually being explored in the area of influencing prevention.[11] It's worth mentioning that although the National Cancer Institute, a branch of the National Institute of Health dedicated to cancer research, does not endorse any dietary supplement aimed at cancer prevention, it does acknowledge garlic as one of the many vegetables out there that have anti-cancer properties; although it is difficult to find the specific amounts needed to decrease cancer risks because of the many varieties and differences available as pertaining to garlic preparations.[12]

There is so much support for my take on eating a wide variety of vegetables. Take advantage of the health benefits they can potentially bring to you and your loved ones, especially, those I personally call "kitchen must-haves". Again, any amount, however little, can count. By all means, cease even those seemingly littlest opportunities. For example, find creative ways to include garlic in some of your recipes when at all possible.

In addition to the many other health benefits, the microbiology in me would not be okay without me mentioning the fact that garlic has been demonstrated to have significant antifungal and antimicrobial properties. Garlic has an ability to inhibit the growth of a range of both Gram-positive and Gram-negative bacteria.[13] Without going into excessive detail, Gram-negative and Gram-positive are two major groupings generally used for differentiating bacteria based on the variations shown in their cell walls, using a type of test known as the Gram stain test. In this test, bacteria are stained using a special "dye". In response to this test, the bacteria would show to be either Gram-positive or Gram-negative. The Gram-positive bacteria have relatively thicker cell walls and retain the color of the "dye", showing a purple coloration when seen under a microscope. On the contrary, Gram-negative bacteria have thin walls and do not retain the dye's color, but reflect a pinkish coloration when observed under a microscope. A substance that has a capability of inhibiting the growth of both Gram-positive and Gram-negative bacteria has a potential of "covering" a wide range of bacteria. This can be of great value to health. Having worked in the area of food microbiology, testing the microbial levels of fresh ready to eat foods, packaged and marketed in grocery stores, I understand what some of these harmful bacteria can do to quickly affect the body internally.

One major thing I love to do as a Biologist and Nurse when taking care of patients with infections, is to look out for any laboratory results that would give an indication of the fact that the growth of bacteria causing certain infections is effectively being inhibited by any treatments my patient may be receiving. Now, you may remember sometimes your doctor has had to change the antibiotics of either you or someone you know during a period of infection, probably because it has not been effective enough in doing its job of inhibiting bacterial growth or, of course, getting rid of them totally. I mention this to let you know that when you come across a vegetable that has great antimicrobial and antifungal activities like garlic, take advantage of it! It could unknowingly save you a few trips to the doctor while actively, or even passively, eating it. Go for it!

I could keep going on and on with the many other amazing properties of garlic that have been shown to be beneficial to boosting the body's health. Hopefully, the few I have mentioned helps to throw light on how beneficial garlic can be to your health. Just to give you an idea of the weight, a clove of garlic from an average bulb could weigh anywhere between 2 and 4 grams. If consumption, greater than 10g daily, has been shown to be effective in decreasing risks of prostate cancer as in the study mentioned above, you'd agree with me that even consumption as low as 1-2 cloves daily in maintaining health could be helpful. As always, little is better than none. The little opportunities you take advantage of can make a big difference in your health.

Slipping garlic-filled recipes into your dietary regimen, even 2-3 times in a week, can be beneficial to your health. If you are fond of some other allium vegetables such as onions, scallions, chives, etc., I say good for you, because eating them can further boost your immune health as well.

For the food in this group (e.g. onions) that can easily be eaten raw, this form of consumption is highly encouraged. Research has pointed to some of the highest benefits from these raw forms of consumption. The next time you prepare your sandwiches at home, or order from a restaurant, be sure not to leave out your onions, as these come as opportunities you can embrace toward simple boosts for your immune system, and your total health at large.

For garlic, both cooked and raw have been shown to be beneficial. As a matter of fact, most people, including myself, consume garlic in cooked form. There are some people who are unable to consume garlic at all in any recipes for various reasons. Garlic comes in supplemental forms as well, and like all other supplements, checking for quality is essential when making purchases of food supplements, and ensuring safety as pertaining to any possible reactions with any prescription medications and allergies. I can't stress enough, the importance of checking with your healthcare provider, most especially whenever you have questions about a new health regimen. By all means, consider adding garlic to your "kitchen must-haves", and your health will thank you.

CHAPTER EIGHTEEN

Cloves

What you do to impact the cells of your
body whether nourishing or intoxicating
them, will go a long way to reflect on
the overall quality of your health.

For many people, cloves typically belong to the group of
spices in the kitchen, generally overlooked and underutilized. Most kitchens have cloves displayed on their spice
racks, and they tend to stay on these racks all year, one year after
the other. There are amazing potential benefits to health that
can be obtained from these cloves that are neatly displayed on
our spice racks. If you haven't already, walk to your spice rack,
read the labels, and try to identify cloves. As you continue to
read, information from this section will help you to carefully
examine and get more familiar with your cloves.

Cloves are harvested from the evergreen tree belonging to the
myrtle family of plants. They have a strong, sweet, aromatic smell,
and are the unopened flower buds of the tree, that have been

dried. The drying process typically results in the hardened spice that shows up in the grocery store. The scientific name for cloves is *Syzygium aromaticum*. Cloves have been said to be native to the Maluku Islands of Indonesia, and popular in some Asian and Eastern African countries such as India, Bangladesh, Tanzania, and Madagascar, where they are commercially harvested.[1] Being an evergreen plant, cloves are obtainable all year round.

Dried cloves are shaped like short nails. You won't miss picking them out in the midst of similar spices if you remember this description. Thankfully, they come with labels in the grocery store. Cloves are typically located in the spice aisles. They come both in whole and ground forms. Storing them at home is very easy, as all you need to do is place them alongside your other spices, either on your spice rack, or wherever you typically store spices. Generally, most containers that are used to package cloves tend to be airtight. Cloves stay well in cool, dry, and dark storage spaces, away from heat and sunlight, and like most spices, stay longer in their airtight containers.

Whenever I buy cloves that happen to be in plastic containers, I prefer to pour them into glass containers that are airtight, and they last a long time for me. Keeping lids tightly closed after use is key to keeping spices' ability to stay full of flavor and effectiveness. Usually, cloves come so dry that I believe the whole ones could last for a year, although I buy them in quantities where I use them within 4-6 months. The ground cloves, I believe, can last about half the duration of the whole ones. The refrigerator would be an even cooler place for storage of your cloves if you tend to buy spices in larger quantities than you typically would need for 4-6 months.

As a rule of thumb, always check the expiratory date on the containers of anything you buy, including spices, as a guide. Always check and read labels to ensure you're buying the purest forms of spices possible, especially noting the list of ingredients. Not only does this help to ensure you obtain the best benefits possible, but it also decreases the chances of consuming possible contaminants.

There are tons of recipes that incorporate the use of cloves. They include sides, entrees, and desserts. The tastes of certain savory and sweet dishes, as well as certain drinks, are enhanced by the aromatic, warm, sweet, flavor of cloves, making cloves a spice with a wide range of uses. Also, keep in mind the fact that because of its intense flavor, all you need is a little to get you the desired flavor, as in most spices. Recipes range from dropping a few cloves in drinks and soups during preparation to making pokes and placing them in meats while cooking along with other spices such as onions, to allow the flavor to infuse into meats.

I hope this gives you a broad idea of some of the various ways cloves are used in the tons of recipes available that incorporate them. Personally, I experiment and try them in various recipes, using both the whole and blended forms. Chai tea is one that uses cloves to bring out its intense, robust, unique flavor. There are many desserts, such as pies and fruit cakes, as well as different types of bread and tons of foods that also credit their special, unique tastes to the incorporation of cloves, from their ingredient list. If you love to explore the health benefits of different plant foods like I do, be sure to consider trying cloves in some of your recipes, and you will not be disappointed. As with all foods, including everything discussed in the book, be sure to watch out for allergies whenever trying foods, especially for the very first time.

Why Cloves?

In ancient times, cloves were among some of the herbs that were used in the treatment of many diseases. Cloves have been known to possess antiseptic, antiviral, antifungal, antibacterial and anti-inflammatory properties. Among many natural products, cloves have been said to be among some of the natural products known to have the highest antioxidant content.[2]

Research studies are ongoing for potentially beneficial natural products, with the aim of finding treatments for cancer. This is due to the fact that many current medical treatments for cancer have been noted to have lots of side effects, many times harmful to the health of patients, and also difficult to bear by patients undergoing such treatments. As though that was not enough, as in the case of many ailments, there is also an evolution along the lines of resistance of some cancer cells to certain anti-cancer medications. These factors and more have fueled a greater quest in research to find a cure for cancer, among natural products.

Cloves have been found via research, to possess outstanding "cell-killing" (cytotoxic) activity toward MCF-7 cells, which are a cell line of human breast cancer cells[3], one of, if not the most studied line of breast cancer cells in history. I mention this, to let you know, and picture, the potential potency of this spice, very often overlooked in our kitchen, but with a high potential ability to make the environments within our bodies difficult for disease to thrive, even tumors.

A study has shown that oleanolic acid, a bioactive component found in a solution of clove extract, while using a solution of ethyl acetate for this extraction, may be effective in treating colorectal cancer.[4] The ethyl acetate extract of cloves in this study has been shown to also inhibit tumor growth and promote cell cycle arrest, as well as cell death or destruction (apoptosis) in certain human cancer cells in various degrees, including breast (MCF-7), ovarian (SKOV-3), cervical

(HeLa), liver (BEL-7402), pancreatic (PANC-1), and colon (HT-29) cells.[5]

Eugenol, a compound found in the oil of cloves and some other aromatic spices, such as cinnamon and basil, have been shown to possess tumor growth suppressing properties.[6] Cloves have been shown to protect the liver. Eugenol extracted from cloves, gives cloves this liver-protective ability, as in the case of liver cirrhosis, in reversing certain changes (biochemical and histopathological changes), and inhibiting the rapid growth (cell proliferation) of these abnormal liver (hepatic) cells.[7]

With its anti-inflammatory properties, imagine the wealth of health benefits that cloves could potentially bring to you. Linking this to the concept of how anti-inflammatories can help boost immune health, think of how a few cloves consumed here and there could help positively impact your health. Cloves, simply extracted in water, have been shown to inhibit inflammation, both acute and chronic as well as inhibit oxidative stress.[8] Recall (from Chapter 3) that oxidative stress can occur in the body when an imbalance is created because the body's rate of production of free radicals is much higher than its ability to counteract, get rid of, or detoxify the harmful effects created by the presence of these free radicals. Foods rich in antioxidant properties are able to neutralize harmful effects from these free radicals, thus, preventing the occurrence of this imbalance that can result in oxidative stress.

We can see that a simple consumption of cloves in our foods can go a long way to help prevent oxidative stress. This goes to further support my advocacy of oral consumption of simple forms of these health-beneficial, immune health-boosting foods such as cloves, in their basic quantities whenever possible, as much as we can, from our everyday food choices. Doing this can go a long way in preventing potential "disruptions" in our health. Remember, what you do to impact the cells of your body whether nourishing or intoxicating them, will go a long way to reflect on the overall quality of your health.

In 2006, a study conducted in Pakistan showed that cloves consumed in various quantities, from 1g to 3g daily for 30 days, improved insulin function in study participants with type 2 diabetes, with serum glucose decreasing from 225+/-67 to 150+/-46 mg/dL.[9] Cholesterol levels in these participants also showed some decrease.[10] The serum glucose level decreases are so significant to me that I thought to mention. This is because the average drop in numbers, using even the high numbers in the range (225 and 150), gives us a difference of 75, which is significant, most especially resulting from consuming such a seemingly simple food. The potential benefits of cloves to improved insulin function is notable and may be well worth this major benefit, while consuming cloves in our foods, especially with a rise of type 2 diabetes in recent times. Just to give you a practical idea of what the weight could be equivalent to, the average weight of a teaspoon of ground spices like cloves is about 2.1grams in weight. In essence, a little goes a long way and would be worth the try.

There are many other beneficial bioactive compounds that have been isolated from cloves other than those mentioned above, as well as flavonoids, that have given cloves so much value in terms of their benefits to health. Cloves can positively impact the digestive and metabolic pathways, and it is no wonder that there are studies that have shown their positive impact on carbohydrate and lipid digestion.[11] As a matter of fact, some of these studies have noted blood glucose-lowering (antihyperglycemic), cholesterol-lowering (antihyperlipidemic), and antioxidant activities in cloves.[12] Clearly, this points to a promising impact of cloves on cholesterol regulation, as well as blood sugar regulation potentials, in the body.

In the dental world, I believe the anti-inflammatory and antibacterial properties of cloves may play a major role for treatment and prevention of gum disease. It is also used effectively in treating bad breath (halitosis).

As you can tell from the discussion, cloves are a valuable spice you can consider placing on your must-have list in your kitchen. It's on mine, and I believe it's worth it. With its load of benefits, a few of which have been highlighted, it is generally considered safe when consumed in the amounts used in foods. In food quantities, the U. S. Food & Drug Administration considers cloves as generally safe.[13] Quantities outside of that have not been certified in terms of safety. For this reason, I'd be very cautious and extremely discretional in the use of clove extracts in oil, and consumption outside of the range of normal food quantities.

Eugenol, one of the health-beneficial bioactive substances in cloves, with its loads of benefits, has also shown a potential to slow down blood clotting.[14] It is important to pay attention to this and consult with your physician if taking medications that cause thinning of your blood such as aspirin, warfarin, etc. From personal experience, I have come to realize that like most foods, consuming cloves and most other spices orally in quantities that do not generally exceed the amounts you would normally put in your foods, tend to be safe. There are many benefits your body can potentially obtain from these amounts. This is worth all the effort of incorporating cloves in your everyday cooking and eating habits. Additionally, like most other spices, cloves have a peculiar taste that can add extra flavor to your cooking.

Typically, it is not easy and simple to go overboard and be excessive in the use of cloves. This is because like most spices, going overboard can make the flavor of your foods come out too strong if it is not intended. Of course, in certain recipes, that may be intended. Believe me, you won't miss the extremes when it comes to adding spices to food. It's like putting excessive sugar in your tea or coffee. The use of even a good thing can be abused if used in excess. However, spices will "shout" at you very easily if you try to go overboard with them.

Practice in usage usually helps with finding the quantities of any spices that are perfect for your foods. The use of cloves is not an exception. As with most things including foods, frequent practice helps you find just the right balance for you. Dare to take the chances you have to boost your immune health via foods like cloves. Start by exploring recipes tried out by others. This can be helpful in aiding you to find your best-preferred quantities.

The most caution I would mention, is in the use of clove oil.[15] Remember, the oil is extracted from the cloves through processes, that have a potential of introducing contaminants, amidst other factors. Use clove oil with extreme caution if ever explored, and refrain from orally giving these oils to children, due to a potential for causing seizures.[16] Once again, this goes to further support my advocacy for oral consumption of these healthful foods such as cloves, in their most natural state and in food-safe quantities.

Consider taking advantage of boosting your immunity and your health at large, by exploring recipes that make use of cloves, and eat them in the amounts you are able to handle. There are so many health benefits of this spice that it would be worth going the extra mile to include in your meals if you are not already doing so.

CHAPTER NINETEEN

Cinnamon

Deliberately find, and at least, occasionally
eat foods that can counteract some of the
potential negative effects from the occasional
consumption of some unhealthy foods.

Cinnamon is a very popular spice in many homes, although many times easily overlooked in terms of its potential health benefits. For many of us, we consume cinnamon in minimum possible quantities, especially in baked goods. Still, other times, many recipes that have cinnamon in them also come intermixed with excessive sugars to such an extent that most of us tend to miss cinnamon's full potential benefits to health.

The everyday cinnamon spice that we have in our kitchens are packaged from the barks of a group of trees, which belong to the scientific genus, *Cinnamomum*. There are several trees from this genus, from which the innermost layers of the barks are harvested, dried, and processed into various forms. These forms eventually make their way from the grocery stores into our homes. There are many delicious savory recipes out there that can be made from cinnamon. When exploring these recipes, try to limit processed sugar or use natural healthy alternatives when possible, so you can truly enjoy and reap the health benefits of cinnamon. If you are open to exploring healthy foods like I am, consider taking advantage of the use of cinnamon in some special dishes. The next time you pick up a cookbook, look out for some of these foods, by searching carefully through the list of ingredients. Consider substitutions of your choice, and experiment with them until you come up with recipes you like.

There are several species of cinnamon, some of the most popular ones being *Cinnamomum cassia* (Chinese cinnamon), *C. verum* (Ceylon or Sri Lanka cinnamon). A distinguishing physical feature between these two popular species, among others, is the fact that Ceylon cinnamon sticks appear to have thinner rolled up layers of bark, as compared to the Cassia whose rolled barks are relatively thicker. The Ceylon appears lighter in color and softer in terms of appearance, having several folds with relatively minimal empty spaces between these folds. I believe this can be attributed to the thinness of its layers. The folds of the Ceylon can be inward or backward, whereas that of the Cassia is typically inward-folding only.

It's important to mention that cinnamon contains coumarin, found in varying quantities in the different species of cinnamon plants. Coumarin has a "blood-thinning" effect, meaning that it can cause an extension of the amount of time needed for blood to clot. If you or anyone you know takes a medication with such effect, some common ones being aspirin and coumadin, you may be familiar with this concept and all the precaution that comes with taking what we commonly call "blood thinners". Don't let this put you off from reaping the potential health benefits of cinnamon, and the reason I say this is that there are tons of common plant foods that contain coumarin. If you are one who consumes cinnamon in significant quantities in your foods, it's important to have knowledge of this. It will come in handy whenever the need arises, so you can work with your healthcare providers to find the right doses of any medications you may be taking that could potentially have similar effects. This is yet another major and important reason to always consult with your healthcare provider, most especially if you are taking any medications for treatment, whenever you start a new regimen.

A major differentiating factor in the species of cinnamon is the relative difference in the levels of coumarin content. Keep in mind that most of the cinnamon spices in our grocery stores do not label the species used, and it is said that most of these are from the Cassia species or mixtures of species[1], which may end up containing high amounts of coumarin. Consuming excessive amounts of coumarin can lead to liver damage.[2] With that said, there is good news for you! This good news is that I outline the differentiating physical appearance of Ceylon. I do this because Ceylon contains very negligible amounts of coumarin, about 250 times less than that of Cassia.[3, 4] I believe this may be the reason Ceylon may be commonly referred to as "true cinnamon", and is mostly preferred over the other varieties. When buying, do what it takes to purchase Ceylon when at all possible, in order to stay on the safer side of use. Remember the physical description of the sticks as a guide.

Cinnamon grows in many different regions and continents including the Caribbean and Asia. The countries Sri Lanka, Indonesia, and China are the highest producers of some of the most widely available commercial forms of cinnamon worldwide. Cinnamon is an evergreen plant, and it's no wonder that it's harvested from a wide variety of countries. The next time you go to the grocery store to buy cinnamon, check your label to see if you can simply find out where it's produced, or the species used. This could even be a fun educational activity for your family, especially kids, as you create innovative ways of getting them involved in making choices for healthy foods, reading labels, and being informed consumers of what they eat.

There is so much "junk" out there competing for the health of our kids, that as a mother and a nurse, given what I see every day, I am passionate about helping families, more so our kids, given their vulnerability, to develop a deep understanding of making healthy picks that will boost their immune health and position them for success in life.

I had to mention this under the section of cinnamon, because this is a spice that most kids naturally develop a liking for, because of its prevalence in a lot of sweet foods. For that reason, it would be a lot easier to find creative ways of getting them to consume more of that in much healthier recipes, including some savory foods, smoothies, and yes, even healthier desserts, while helping them enjoy their way up the ladder of health.

In the grocery store, cinnamon can be found both in the ground form, as well as in the stick form. Typically, they are located in the spices aisle and produced by a wide range of brands. It's interesting to state that because cinnamon sticks have some uses in craft, they are also found in lots of craft stores, where they tend to be cheaper compared to those we buy from the grocery store. However, lots of those for craft are not prepared for consumption. It's important to keep that in mind whenever you plan on making any edible craft activities involving the use of cinnamon. Be careful to buy those prepared specifically for eating, with typically minimal potential "contaminants" in comparison to the solely craft-prepared ones.

Some people needing the ground forms of cinnamon prefer to buy the sticks and grind them, mostly using a coffee grinder. I must say that hot cocoa tastes wonderful with some ground cinnamon added, a quick home tip for the whole family. It's fun to buy organic sticks and grind them at home if you can. In addition to saving some money, it also gets you more flavor in its use. Keep in mind that for the reasons previously outlined, always go for Ceylon. Buying them in sticks will help you better identify Ceylon and help you to avoid excessive consumption of coumarin from cinnamon while obtaining its health benefits.

The amazing thing about spices is, they seem to last forever, and you can attest to this by visiting your spice rack. I have realized from my personal experiences though it's important to be careful to note the decrease in potency of the flavors over time, to know when they need to be replaced. Doing this will help you to get the most benefit out of your spices, for your health. Keep this in mind, especially if you happen to buy spices that do not display expiratory dates. As with most other foods however, use the expiratory date displayed on your container as additional guide if available, whenever you purchase cinnamon. I have seen ground cinnamon last as long as a little over 6 months past the expiratory date, and its sticks averaging 2 years on the shelf.

As in most if not all foods, the fresher you have them, the better they are for you and your health. Cinnamon is no exception, and its potency generally begins to decrease following the manufacturer's displayed expiratory date. In order to maintain the potency of cinnamon, it is best to store cinnamon in a container with a close-fitting, tight lid, and keep in a kitchen cabinet (or wherever you typically keep your spices), preferably in a cool, dry, dark, place, away from sunlight, and of course, heat.

Why Cinnamon?

Cinnamon is a spice that has been around for a long time. It continues to baffle many for its outstanding benefits. Health communities continue to unearth rewards from the consumption of cinnamon. Some of the bioactive substances that give cinnamon its health benefits include cinnamaldehyde, eugenol, and camphor, found in various parts of the plant, in varying quantities.[5] There are tons of research studies that point to cinnamon as having properties that are of great benefit to our health.

Lots of research has been done using various species of cinnamon, many of which focus on *Cinnamomum cassia,* and *Cinnamomum verum* (Ceylon cinnamon). I believe these are widely explored because of the more common commercial availability of *C. cassia;* and in the case of *C. verum,* its relatively negligible content of coumarin compared to its other common cassia species counterpart, making it a relatively safer choice, especially for people who consume cinnamon in comparatively higher amounts than the average person.

Outside of the safety concerns of high coumarin levels in *C. cassia,* both of these popular species have proven beneficial to the body. Keep in mind that Ceylon cinnamon is named after the former name of Sri Lanka (Ceylon), the country of its origin. Up until recently, Ceylon cinnamon was scientifically called *Cinnamomum zeylanicum*[6], and you would thus find some literature referencing it as such. Hopefully, all these highlights will help you to remember to look for Ceylon cinnamon, the safer kind of cinnamon.

Among the many health benefits noted from cinnamon, it is worth mentioning its potential ability in lowering blood glucose, blood pressure, and cholesterol, as well as its ability to work against certain parasites and bacteria, and its potential ability to prevent the formation of certain Alzheimer's disease markers (tau aggregation and filament formation); its potential wound-healing benefits, as well as its potential liver protection benefits[7], just to highlight a few.

Cinnamon's ability to boost your immune health can further be seen from its ability to scavenge free radicals (Chapter 3) and its ability to act as an antioxidant.[8] It is easy to see how these properties can help boost your immune health, from the understanding of some of the concepts extensively discussed earlier. This is the reason I place cinnamon as one of my special spices, particularly, Ceylon cinnamon. It's worth considering on your list also.

With the rise in cases of newly diagnosed type 2 diabetes cases, prevention, most importantly through lifestyle and dietary measures is one of the best gifts anyone can give to themselves and their loved ones. This is because, from my professional and everyday interactions with people, I have come to find out that one of the key factors that have contributed immensely to the increase in type 2 diabetes, and which is typically preventable but generally overlooked, is the increase in sedentary lifestyle (lack of activity) and unhealthy eating habits in our communities today.

I have previously outlined tips that will help you keep up with your body's essential needs in the fast-paced world we live in today. Consider foods like cinnamon valuable, as they can help to boost the body's immune health, and which in turn, can help the body to cope with the demands of life. Like most research, a few studies of cinnamon, have not found proven benefits in blood sugar-lowering capabilities. Yet, of significant importance is the fact that there are lots of other studies showing cinnamon to be of benefit to lowering blood sugar levels.

Again, this goes a long way to support my statement that different foods may work differently for different people. Trying until you find what is just right for you is worth it, given that there are a wide variety of foods with similar health benefits. Additionally, eating a wide variety of health-beneficial foods is always an advantage when it comes to boosting your health. In so doing you get a correspondingly wide range of benefits while decreasing any potential downsides that could result from over-consumption of even a good thing. With that said, there have been studies that have pointed to a positive effect of cinnamon on blood sugar regulation.

A study in China showed an improvement in fasting blood sugar levels and Hemoglobin A1c levels of patient study participants who consumed various amounts of cinnamon daily (some 120 milligrams, others 360 milligrams), as against the study group that did not consume cinnamon (placebo).[9] Measurements of the Hemoglobin A1c and fasting blood sugar levels are commonly used in assessing the effectiveness of the body's ability to regulate its blood sugar levels and are common assessments you'd come across, most especially with diabetics. There are several studies that support the positive effect of cinnamon on blood sugar regulation, and many studies have also demonstrated this ability, using laboratory animals[10, 11], as is usually the case in lots of research, especially at the initial phase of exploration.

Of equally great significance is a cholesterol-lowering ability of cinnamon, shown with some studies carried out to find its ability to improve blood sugar levels.[12, 13] In decreasing total cholesterol, it's worth mentioning the fact cinnamon has been shown to have the ability to both increase the body's levels of good cholesterol/ fat (High-Density Lipoprotein), as well as decrease levels of bad cholesterol/fat (Low- Density Lipoprotein).[14] This is a great factor worth mentioning. Remember, in the discussion of fats (also see Chapter 10), we outlined the importance of making sure we consume foods that help to increase our body's levels of "good fats" (which our bodies need for healthy function), while decreasing the consumption of foods high in "bad fats". A good balance of these two phenomena will better equip the body in ensuring that it has a healthy overall total cholesterol management, with high levels of the good (HDL), and low levels of the bad (LDL).

I mentioned the significance of sources of fats from plant foods, as being a valuable way of obtaining "good fats". Plant-derived fats can afford the body the capability to achieve its healthy objective of maintaining high levels of "good fats". On the contrary, decreasing the consumption of fats from animal foods, would help to decrease the levels of "bad fats". Cinnamon, although not a source of fat in comparison to plant foods that have high sources of fats, as in avocado, etc., has a potential ability to fuel the body to achieve this objective of healthy fat regulation. I believe even better results can be realized when combined with eating the right kinds of fat as described.

Cinnamon has been found to have the ability to counteract some of the potential negative effects that result from eating a high fructose or high-fat diet.[15] These negative effects could be that on behavior, the brain's signals pertaining to the action of insulin, as well as Alzheimer's-related changes.[16] With cinnamon's ability to influence the brain's actions on its insulin-regulating function, it is no wonder that certain type 2 diabetics have realized an improved insulin regulation and better blood sugar control from simply eating cinnamon.

It's important to note that initially in most research studies (especially in health-related research studies when it involves testing a drug or food substance's effect on the health of the body), laboratory animals are used. Safety and ethical concerns of using humans in studies especially when outcomes are uncertain and possible complications are unknown, leads researchers to manipulate experimental features being tested (variables) in laboratory animals. Ideas are tested out until it's typically determined safe to test in humans. Without going into extreme details, I can tell you this has led to lots of breakthrough studies, which allow us to enjoy better health today.

When it comes to foods, we eat quantities we know to be safe. It is important to know most of these tests are carried out to find their health benefits at higher intake. However, they provide significant information that helps us know how our health is impacted by our food choices. I am saying this to support the fact that if you know the potential benefits of some of these foods to your health as in the case of cinnamon and many others, it may be necessary to educate yourself about how to safely find pure forms of them and eat in normal food quantities to reap benefits from them. It's worth considering using some of these "health-full" foods to boost your immune health.

Cinnamon extract has been shown to have a capacity of suppressing the growth of tumor cells.[17] Cinnamon is able to stimulate tumor cells to die by interacting with certain key factors that naturally play a role in promoting the growth of tumor cells.[18, 19] Researchers point to this ability as a potential for exploration, in the area of treating tumors. We know cancer cells typically form from tumors. Hence, we can infer a key potential benefit of cinnamon here, to health. This information goes to further support the value of this amazing kitchen spice.

Its capability of potentially suppressing the growth of tumor cells can contribute to cinnamon's ability to create an "environment" in your body that makes it difficult for unwanted "organisms" to thrive. Such environments can make it difficult for "harmful organisms", or even certain "abnormal cell growths" to thrive and perpetuate, thus, contributing to strengthening the immune system (Refer to Chapter 8). This is in alignment with the key concepts discussed earlier about making "your swimming pool" a fabulous one, to give your health a boost.

With the current trends in diet and the many negative effects to health that sometimes come along with frequently eating unhealthy foods, I personally love to deliberately find, and at least, occasionally eat foods that can counteract some of the potential negative effects from some of these unhealthy foods. This is an approach I believe should be considered, as it can be a plus to boosting the body's immune health, in our pursuit of optimal health. I am glad to say that cinnamon is one that can potentially help in this aspect of wellness.

Many ready-to-eat, store-bought foods and snacks contain immense quantities of high fructose corn syrup and significant amounts of "bad fats". It is needful to have knowledge of some of these kitchen essentials that can be useful in counteracting some potential effects from the occasional consumption of such foods. Keep in mind, success is realized from minimal consumption of these, and strive for consuming healthy foods at least 85% of your overall weekly intake, as discussed in Chapter 8. Additionally, an ability of cinnamon to protect nerve cells from damage, degeneration, or "malfunction" (neuroprotective effects) can be seen in its capability of counteracting some of the potentially negative effects that pertain to Alzheimer's-related changes in the brain[20] as mentioned earlier. Some of these negative effects can be potentially triggered by the consumption of large amounts of "bad fats" and high fructose corn syrup from diets. Frequent consumption can add up too. Thus, cinnamon's ability to positively impact the brain's health is a plus. Alzheimer's is on the rise, and many pointers to possible causes are being researched, including diet-related causes.

Making healthy changes to your diet can be valuable in possible prevention, and your occasional cinnamon consumption could further boost this effort. I could keep going with many other potential benefits of cinnamon, including an ability to positively aid the body in blood pressure regulation (an antihypertensive effect).[21] Cinnamon's antioxidant property[22, 23] is worth mentioning, as this can help with it enabling the body to counteract the potentially harmful effect of free radicals (see Chapter 3). Foods with antioxidant properties are priceless when it comes to boosting our immune health. It's very important to include them in our dietary regimen.

As from our discussions of major concepts and their application, the use of *"tactful" moderation* is key to obtaining maximum benefits from your spices. You can benefit from the application of this concept in the consumption of cinnamon. Eating a variety of health-beneficial foods is essential to boosting your immune health. Consider adding cinnamon to your options. Keep in mind the discussion of varying levels of coumarin in various species of cinnamon when making your selections. Go for Ceylon species whenever it's within your power to do so. Be watchful of any potential allergies, most especially when trying foods for the first time. Be sure to check with your physician for any potential interactions with treatments or your current medications. With all these potential benefits of cinnamon in mind, consider including it on your list of kitchen favorites so you can obtain the benefits it can potentially bring to boosting your health.

CHAPTER TWENTY

The Mint Family

Consider taking them off display and décor
mode on your kitchen countertop, to an action
and health-boosting mode in your body.

This family of plants, scientifically known as Lamiaceae, is notable, in that it has lots of members that are useful in our kitchens as herbs for seasoning lots of our foods. More so, these herbs are loaded with great potential benefits to health. Their fragrance and/or flavor-enhancing features make them popular in our kitchens. Just to name a few, you may be familiar with thyme, basil, oregano, marjoram, sage, and mint. All of these belong to this family of plants, even the lavender plant.

I chose to discuss only a few of these plants because I want to make it easy to connect their benefits to health. These selected few I focus on also tend to be common in most kitchens, although many times severely underutilized. My goal is to outline some of the benefits these few I highlight can potentially bring to you in boosting your immune health so you can begin to consider mindfully including at least some of them in your cooking and dietary regimen.

The great news is, some of these bioactive substances that provide these health benefits tend to be found in varying quantities across the different plants from the family. Thus, the more from the variety you can creatively consume or use from this family of plants, the more benefits you can potentially obtain from them. The wonderful thing about these is that because they each possess a unique robust flavor and smell, it can be simple and easy to purposefully get creative with their use and consumption, while obtaining benefits from them, in boosting your health. Some people try to eat certain ones occasionally but may not realize the importance of finding ways of maximizing consumption for the benefit of their body's health.

Strong anti-inflammatory, antioxidant, and antibacterial properties tend to run common in many plants from this family. This makes them invaluable for boosting the body's immune health. As you read on, you may realize the need to take them off display and décor mode on your kitchen countertop, to an action and health-boosting mode in your body, if you are not already doing so. I can tell you from many experiences, you can use these to your advantage, and I hope after reading about these, you are able to visualize some of the potential benefits these plants can bring to your own health. Most importantly, I hope you can consider beginning to explore recipes and other means of using some plants from this family, in boosting your immune health, and of course, your overall health.

Rosemary

If you are a lover of plants and tend to grow edible potted plants in your home, or even tend to take a special look at them in pots when you see them in the produce aisle while visiting the grocery store, you most likely have come across, or are familiar with the rosemary plant. The scientific name of this plant is *Rosmarinus officinalis.* The Rosemary plant can live for more than two years, and belongs to the category of plants known as perennials. This plant is evergreen and has a distinguishing feature of needle-like leaves when compared to similar plants. It belongs to a large family of flowering plants scientifically known as Lamiaceae[1], and commonly referred to as the mint family, as just introduced.

Rosemary is cultivated in various regions of the world, across various continents. It tends to flourish in warmer environmental conditions. Rosemary grows both outdoors, and indoors in potted plants. When grown outdoors and even indoors, it can form a thick "bush" and is able to do well even in winter conditions, when kept together with other potted plants indoors. This makes it one of the favorites for gardeners who also like to keep indoor plants.

In the grocery store, rosemary is most commonly sold in small potted plants, or even as simple twigs with its leaves, when you want to buy them fresh somehow. It can also be bought in dried packaged forms in the spice aisle. For those who love to cook, I hope you've tried some of the amazing culinary uses of rosemary, as it has a unique flavor that can further enhance your cooking, whether it's in meats in your pot roasts, or even vegetables when baking or stir-frying. Again, there are tons of recipes out there that explore the culinary uses of rosemary, and I can tell you they're worth every try. If you love its flavor, consider tweaking more of your favorite recipes to promote more rosemary consumption.

Storing rosemary is simple. In the fresh forms, I have stored them for up to about 2 weeks in the vegetable tray of my refrigerator, in simple vegetable bags from the grocery store. Freezing excess rosemary makes it easy to get a hold of "semi-fresh" forms as I call this form, when I need fresh substitutes for cooking. I have used this form as far as 3 months and sometimes a little beyond, and it has stayed well for me. Storing rosemary in a dry spice form follows the usual convention for storing dry spices, and they typically last long, as with many other spices. Checking for flavor is key to knowing when it's time to throw out that unused spice, especially if you do not see any expiratory date on the packaging container. Store your dried spice in a dry, cool, and dark place, usually a cabinet where you typically store your other spices, away from sunlight and heat. This can help it stay potentially for up to about 2-3 years. Be sure to check expiratory dates if available.

People who grow rosemary at home are able to air dry and have this wonderful herb dry completely. They are then able to keep these dry forms in airtight containers for about a few weeks to a couple of months if completely dried with no moisture, like you see packaged at the grocery store. Your choices of how to keep yours would typically depend on the recipes you like, and the forms in which you need rosemary in these recipes, whether fresh or dry. You have options. Make your picks.

I like to have both forms, and it works perfectly for me. When you are selecting your rosemary, like all your other spices, you should look out for its appearance and quality. Rosemary extracts in the form of essential oils are also available on the market. Also, keep quality at heart whenever you purchase these. It would be helpful to keep these in mind, as you explore rosemary-rich recipes and various other uses of rosemary in boosting your health.

Why Rosemary?

Rosemary has amazing benefits to health. Just to whet your appetite, let me give you a brief overview of a group of residents who live in Acciaroli, Italy, from a story, highlighted in the New York Times.[2] In this city, the average number of older residents at the age of 90 or older is higher (about one in every 60), as compared to most regions around the world. Of great significance is the lifestyle of this senior population, in comparison to the rest of the world. In fact, the lifestyle of this special group of people has become an attraction for researchers, most especially their condition of good health, even at age 90 and beyond.[3] The abundance of rosemary in this region of the world, most especially, a very potent species, and its high use among this population, has become a major factor of interest, and researchers point to this as one of the possible factors that enhance longevity in this group of residents.[4] Rosemary has been found to have immense benefits to human health, and I believe it is no wonder that this group of residents who consume so much of it, experience such great health and longevity. As I discuss some of the benefits of rosemary to health, I'll make occasional references to these residents, so you can make a seamless mental connection to some of these potential health benefits when you personally consume rosemary.

There are various bioactive compounds that give rosemary its health benefits, and of significance is the group known as the phenolic diterpenes (such as carnosic acid and carnosol), because of the wide range of health benefits attributable to them.[5] Rosmarinic acid gives rosemary its antioxidant property.[6]

A wide range of health benefits are attributable to rosemary, and these include an ability to fight certain bacteria (antimicrobial), anti-inflammatory, antioxidant, as well as cancer-fighting (anti-cancer or anti-carcinogenic) and liver protecting (hepatoprotective) properties.[7] The liver is the major organ in our body that helps with removal of toxic substances from within, and thus, protecting this organ is highly important to the function of the body. The bioactive compounds carnosic acid and carnosol (accounting for over 90% of rosemary's benefits), have been said to be major contributors of the plant's anti-inflammatory, antioxidant, anti-carcinogenic and neuroprotective (protects nerve cells, as in those found in the brain) benefits.[8]

Of great significance is the potential benefit of rosemary to the health of brain cells, as shown in its neuroprotective properties.[9, 10] The increase in certain brain-related diseases in our society today like Parkinson's and Alzheimer's have become a great concern to many. The absolute cause of these is many times unknown. Finding foods that could potentially help keep the health of brain cells up high while potentially avoiding some of these diseases is very needful. Rosemary can be of great benefit to people with Alzheimer's and Parkinson's. The reason for this is, extracts from rosemary have been found to have an ability to act as protectants of brain cells while also preventing the action of agents that influence brain cell death.[11, 12] The protective properties of extracts from the leaves of this amazing plant on brain cells are further enhanced by its anti-inflammatory[13] and antioxidant effects, making it a real "jewel" to brain health. This potential brain health benefit can further be supported by the lives of the senior citizen residents of Acciaroli, Italy. Not only do they live so long, but they are seen to be mentally active even in their old age, with a low incidence of Alzheimer's disease.[14] In fact, it is said of these residents that at age 95, an average individual's brain function is equivalent to that of a 50-year-old[15]. This is very impressive. Its anti-inflammatory and antioxidative properties further lend rosemary an edge in being beneficial to heart health (cardiovascular health)[16] as well.

In addition to the flavor rosemary can add to your cooking, it can also help you better enjoy your red meat the next time you eat it. Whether it's from beans, or fruits and vegetables, including more plants in your dietary regimen can be very helpful in boosting your immune health. Eating fish, chicken, and beef, with the right amount, frequency, and quality in mind, is equally important. This is because each of these bring essential benefits to health if eaten right. Generally, I like to keep beef to once or twice a week, making sure I eat more of green leafy vegetables along with my other protein sources to ensure I get sufficient iron intake. Particularly on days when I eat fish or chicken, I try to pay attention to increasing my green leafy vegetables. I also closely intersperse those days with days of dark poultry consumption, with the *concept of balance* in mind. I am able to maintain good iron levels for many weeks without red meat consumption whenever I choose to, by simply eating reasonable amounts of dark meat chicken and turkey, along with some of the mentioned green leafy vegetables. I find that very helpful. I hope you find these helpful when planning meals for yourself or your loved ones.

Some people choose to avoid beef altogether due to certain concerns, and that's alright, especially if they are ensuring adequate intake of iron-rich foods from other sources such as the green leafy vegetable group, beets, and much more. Buying minimally processed beef from sources where animals are not hormone fed is ideal whenever possible, for those of us who enjoy its benefits occasionally. However, these tend to be expensive. Additionally, many people mentally battle with the possibility of consuming potentially harmful substances (heterocyclic amines), known to be formed when meat is cooked at high temperatures. For this reason, there are many who shy away from consuming red meats totally.

I have good news for you, if this is a concern for you but you enjoy the occasional consumption of red meat, once or sometimes twice some weeks. Studies using beef patties have shown that rosemary extracts are able to decrease the formation of these potentially harmful substances (heterocyclic amines), produced when beef is cooked at high heat, by as much as a 90% decrease in its formation.[17] Hopefully, this will help you to be able to better introduce occasional meat consumption in your diet with confidence, as you "slap" lots of rosemary on your meat, whether grilling or simply steaming. If these potential body toxins have been a concern for you in the past, try rosemary. This is a double win, as you get to enjoy the taste of your food while reaping the health benefits of rosemary in the process. Like most foods, even a little goes a long way once it gets into the body. Do you see why rosemary made it to the list of my kitchen must-haves? I hope you consider putting this on yours also.

The list gets even better and fancier. Like its sister herb from the same family, Lavender, the simple inhalation of the fragrance of rosemary from its essential oil forms, has been shown to stimulate positive activity in both the brain and nervous system, with an ability to enhance mood.[18] Rosemary has been shown to be potentially beneficial to eye health, as pertaining to age-related changes to the eye, and this benefit explored in combination with other substances.[19]

Many natural beauty products explore the benefits of rosemary both for the aroma and the benefits it can give to hair and skin. I am an ardent fan of these, and I do my best to use some of these natural products to my benefit and to the benefit of my loved ones. The next time you read labels on your natural skin products, look out for rosemary.

The bioactive substances in rosemary have been shown to possess anti-cancer properties.[20] With so much fight for life in the area of cancer, I realize the need to highlight some of these foods that are rich in polyphenols and other bioactive substances, and which can potentially add to making the environment in our bodies difficult for even potential cancer cells to thrive and propagate themselves, while boosting our immune health.

With some of the great potential health benefits possessed by rosemary, considering this spice/herb with such versatility of use on your list of kitchen must-haves, is worth every effort. Keep in mind as you do this, that like any plant foods, growing processes and conditions can enhance or decrease levels of nutrients in herbal plants. Rosemary is no exception to this rule. For this reason, keeping quality at heart when purchasing rosemary is essential, so you can maximally enjoy its potential benefits to your health.

Thyme

Thyme is another wonderful evergreen perennial, belonging to the nutrition-rich family Lamiaceae, as mentioned earlier. It has the scientific name *Thymus*, with the species *Thymus vulgaris* being the most common. Like rosemary, thyme is another popular culinary spice, also explored in ornamental use. Its relatively smaller leaves and thin stem provide distinguishing features that come in handy for identification.

As in rosemary, commercially available forms of thyme include dry, fresh, essential oil forms, as well as in assorted mixtures with other herbs. Buying and storing of fresh and dry forms also follow the same format as rosemary. Having reviewed that of rosemary, I believe you are well positioned to handle your thyme in some of the best ways possible. Of significance also is the unique aromatic flavor thyme can add to enhance tastes in cooking. It serves really well in many Italian dishes, and seasons meats very well. Explore and try out some recipes with thyme. As in many spices, thyme can be used in combination with other spices, such as rosemary, cloves, and much more, depending on your desired resulting flavors and tastes.

Among the various bioactive substances in thyme, some of the major compounds worth mentioning are carvacrol, and thymol. There are lots of medications and substances that are produced in the chemical and pharmaceutical industry that are manufactured in large quantities from the initial study of potent and beneficial bioactive compounds in certain plants. Scientific study of the chemical structures of some of these plant-derived bioactive substances has become a bedrock that has led to the successful manufacturing in large quantities of some of the most useful substances in the chemical and pharmaceutical industries. I'm mentioning this at this time because thymol is so common on the market that it would be easy to use it in enhancing this understanding of the production of certain helpful substances from the study of the chemical structures of some useful plant-based compounds.

Furthermore, these kinds of scientific studies continue to advance, and who knows where these will lead, as in breakthroughs for combating certain chronic diseases, and cancers. This is the reason I am a firm believer we need to pay attention to research findings and possible clues, that can help to promote health naturally. This forms the foundation for the reason why I provide relevant notes to certain scientific studies throughout the book. I only mention a few out of the volumes of studies that have been done, to help you make simple connections and discover ways in which you can increase your health by what you eat and do.

Now back to thymol. If you like to use certain mouthwashes like Listerine, and many over the counter products, you must have come across thymol. On the market, thymol-containing products usually come in combinations with various other oils and flavors from other plants of this family and still others, like mint, eucalyptus, just to name a few. The next time you buy products, look out for thymol. Thymol is naturally occurring in thyme. The use of thymol in lots of products like mouthwashes stems from its ability to fight bacteria. Thyme has strong antimicrobial activities, attributable to its rich flavonoid content.[1] In fact, thymol and carvacrol from thyme have been shown to decrease the resistance of certain bacteria to certain antibiotic medications like ampicillin, penicillin, tetracycline, bacitracin, erythromycin, and novobiocin.[2] This is great, as this finding could lead to a future of making certain antibiotics more effective against bacteria, especially those that have grown resistant to "treatments" over time.

The antimicrobial effect of thyme is sometimes explored in its use sometimes as a preservative in the food industry. Thyme extracts have been shown to be effective against certain food-related bacteria and fungi.[3] Thyme extracts have been shown to be effective against many bacteria, as well as *Candida albicans*[4], a naturally occurring yeast in the gastrointestinal tract and various parts of the body, also responsible for the cause of the most common yeast infections in the body.

Yeast infections generally occur when yeast's normal balance in the body is offset by certain unusual conditions, and it increases in numbers above the body's normal levels. For ladies with painful menstruation, also known as dysmenorrhea, it may be helpful to know about a study using extracts from the popular species of thyme (*T. vulgaris*) on participants with this condition. Thyme was found to be as effective as ibuprofen (a popular painkiller) in reducing the spasm and pain that comes with this condition.[5]

Polyphenol-rich extracts from a wild species of thyme have shown protective effects of thyme against oxidative stress and hypertension.[6] Extracts from *T. vulgaris,* referred to as naringenin, has been shown to have an ability to inhibit the growth of human colorectal and breast cancer cells, and also make these cells more sensitive to chemotherapy treatment.[7]

Like some of the health-beneficial kitchen must-haves previously discussed, thyme has a great potential to positively influence the treatment of certain conditions in the near future. Dermatologists continue to explore anti-inflammatory and antibacterial properties in treating acne. A study has been carried out using a skin cream mixture containing 3% thyme essential oil. Results from this study showed a 66.5% success of complete healing from acne using the 3% thyme essential oil extract, as compared to the use of non-thyme containing mixes.[8]

Like most of the foods discussed, consuming and using thyme in quantities you would usually use or consume in food is your safest way of getting the best out of this great "healthfull" spice. Be very cautious in uses outside of this zone, as too much of even a good thing, could be harmful to the body. Avoid orally consuming forms that are not meant for that purpose, as in essential oil forms commercially available. Always read labels and follow directions, if choosing to go outside of normal food quantity consumption amounts and forms, of any spices or foods.

Keep in mind that outside of food quantities, active ingredients, including thymol could get out of control from the amounts your body can potentially handle. Be safe, consider getting thyme on your must-have list in your kitchen. As for potentially over consuming when added to your foods, don't worry about that. This is because when excessively added to foods, spices have a way of "speaking up", and will let you know right away, leaving little room for you to go overboard with them. Initially, it will be helpful to follow measurements from new recipes until you get used to estimating amounts you enjoy best. Consider consuming thyme normally in food quantities and enjoy its potential benefits to your health.

Oregano

For most of us, the mention of oregano may remind us of our visit to our favorite sub restaurants. Yes, that spice you are offered at the deli, and have sprinkled on your sandwich could make a wealth of difference in your health. It sure enhances the taste of the sub sandwich, and if you are like me, it can become one of your favorite seasonings for your sub.

The scientific name for oregano is *Origanum vulgare,* also belonging to the family Lamiaceae (most commonly known as the mint family). Are you familiar with marjoram? It's usually a component of lots of dry Italian spices and also poultry seasonings on the market. Marjoram is one of the several varieties of oregano. The next time you shop for some of your favorite herbal spice mixes, read the label to see what you find as pertaining to labeling for oregano, and marjoram.

Commercially available forms of oregano, buying, and storage of dry and fresh forms, follow the same in the family, as in that described for rosemary. Like most of its counterparts in the family, oregano serves many culinary uses, of which I hope you are enjoying or hopefully, considering exploring. Oregano is commonly used in combination with others in its family, and still others outside of its family, in the creation of amazing herbal spices. Oregano has many properties in common with some of the members of its family. As with thyme, oregano has phenolic compounds, with major ones being thymol and carvacrol.

These substances attribute to oregano, some of its great potential health benefits. Extracts from oregano have been shown to have antioxidant, antibacterial, and "cell-killing" (cytotoxic, a property used in this context, usually explored in treating cancer cells) properties.[1]

Having mentioned some of the potential health benefits of thymol and carvacrol, this is a good time to say, that it is worth the little extras from more foods like oregano. In fact, combinations from some of these herbs from this family of plants not only enhance the flavor of your food but can enhance your health as well. To further support this statement, let me mention that the ability of rosemary (discussed under Rosemary) to decrease the release of potentially harmful substances (heterocyclic amines) released when beef is cooked under high temperatures, has also been found to be present in oregano. As mentioned earlier, these substances (heterocyclic amines) have been noted to have a potentially negative impact on the health of the body. However, combining rosemary and oregano can further increase the concentration of rosmarinic acid, making a spice mixture polyphenol-rich.[2] Adding a polyphenol-rich spice like a mixture of rosemary and oregano to hamburger meat before cooking has been shown to decrease the amount of potentially "health-harmful" substances (heterocyclic amines) produced when beef is exposed to high temperatures during cooking.[3]

Adding this simple step to your cooking can make a wealth of difference in your health by decreasing your potential intake of some of these potentially harmful substances, often classified as potential carcinogens (substances that have an ability to start the formation of cancer cells in a living tissue). Oregano has been shown to retain its strong antioxidant properties both in fresh and dry forms.[4] This is very important, as it can help in increasing your confidence in the fact that whatever form you choose to consume oregano, whether dry or fresh, you are making a difference in your health.

In healthcare today, there is an increasing concern over growing ineffectiveness of certain treatments against some "strong" bacteria. For example, MRSA (methicillin-resistant *Staphylococcus aureus*) has evolved resistance to certain medications over time. There is a huge need for alternatives that would help in successfully treating infections from some of these organisms that have developed resistance to certain treatments. In the hospital, workers have to dress up in protective gear to prevent the spread of some of these infectious bacteria when anticipating coming into contact with a patient suffering from an infection from such bacteria as MRSA. They are difficult to treat, and we try to do our best to prevent spreading them. These drug-resistant organisms continue to evolve.

Strong antimicrobial properties of oregano in essential oil extract form, has been shown to be effective against Multidrug-Resistant Bacterial Strains (such as MRSA), with an even higher effectiveness against these bacteria when combined with biological silver nanoparticles.[5] Results from this study indicate that this mixture can potentially provide an approach to taking care of infections that have not responded well to current treatment.[6] That's how potent oregano is, and I state these to bring out its potential benefit to your health when you consume it.

Among many other uses, a few drops of essential oils from aromatic herbs such as oils prepared from plants from the mint family (e.g. oregano, rosemary, mint, etc.) when put in hot water and inhaled, has been shown to be effective in treatment of certain Upper Respiratory Tract Infections (URTIs)[7], like the common cold. Antimicrobial and antiviral properties from some of these oils make them potent against some of these infections. Commercially available essential oils from oregano also come in combinations with those from various other plants, both from the mint family, as well as from others, like eucalyptus. It's amazing the quick relief some of these oils can bring to nasal congestion. These can come in very handy, especially in the winter months, while also eating healthy to boost your immune health.

The strong antioxidant property shown by oregano[8], has a corresponding strong potential to boost your immune health. As you continue to eat your fruits and vegetables, consider also including some of these great herbs in your diet. Together, they will go a long way in adding those extra strides necessary for boosting your immune health.

I hope these highlights have created a desire to explore the many more health benefits that oregano and other members of the mint family can bring to your health. As always, keep in mind the need to buy high-quality forms when shopping for these spices and/or herbs, and consume them in normal food quantities, looking out for any allergies whenever trying any foods for the first time. I hope you've been challenged to consider adding oregano to your list of kitchen must-haves, if you have not already done so.

CHAPTER TWENTY-ONE

Teas From Your Kitchen

*Your health is your most valuable asset,
and it's worth making every effort necessary
to take good care of it. You can train your
taste buds to align with your health goals.*

There are many health-beneficial herbal spices in our kitchen that are also available in tea forms. Many of these are from the Lamiaceae plant family. For example, rosemary and thyme leaves are available and can be brewed in tea forms. There are some people who enjoy drinking teas and can use this like for teas to boost their immune health. Yes, those herbal teas can make a difference! Take advantage of them. Various parts of these great herbal plants, most commonly the leaves, are dried and packaged into tea bag forms. There are still other tea forms, where you can simply put in coffee filters in small preferred amounts, pour hot boiling water over, and allow to steep for about 15 to 20 minutes, after which you can strain and drink. I enjoy the various forms. Like any foods, putting measures in place to buy high-quality forms of herbal teas should be as important as the desire to reap benefits from any you want to try, at any given time.

I grew up seeing my dad, a German-educated physician, using some of these teas successfully in treating certain health conditions. In some cases, success stories included canceling certain scheduled surgical procedures for some of his patients, because they were willing to try, and responded well from drinking certain teas. There are many herbs that date back centuries in terms of discovery, especially in Europe. With modernization, some of these very beneficial herbs have become underutilized, although in ancient times those were all they had most times, and they were successful in treating certain debilitating conditions with them.

With current dietary trends and the continual evolution of the modern diet, many people continue to miss out on the potential benefits of certain key plants to health. My heart goes out most especially to our younger generation who have not heard of, or experienced some of these benefits. There are so many diseases that we see in children these days that were rare in kids a few years back. Sadly enough, society does not do much to encourage healthy eating habits in kids, especially in the area of including plant foods in their diet. There are current attempts to help to improve that, but we still have a long way to go, when kids' menus in lots of restaurants are specially tailored to exclude vegetables.

It's important to eat with potential health benefits in mind, and not only for taste. Of equal importance, let's teach our children this principle by example. It can help prevent them from having to deal with certain conditions such as obesity and other chronic diseases in their near future. By all means, enjoy those occasional treats. In applying the *85:15 concept* for kids, this is where parents can give kids at least a 75% to 80% of healthy meals, while they keep theirs above 85%. This is because kids at a tender, growing, age, have a slightly stronger capability within their bodies to buffer "junk" in comparison to adults, especially if they are active kids who burn lots of calories. Generally, this capability stays until they get into their mid to late teenage years, when it becomes necessary to adjust ratios to fit more closely to their lifestyles, as in adults. This ratio refers to that of healthy versus unhealthy foods, and not calories. Calories should always be tailored to meet an individual's personal requirement, based on generally acceptable guides (use dependable resources, as in that previously mentioned from choosemyplate.gov).

Moderation is still highly encouraged in our younger age groups, as they tend to consume "junk" a little more frequently than the average adult. Excesses in "junk" consumption are still discouraged, as these can take a toll on the body, whether it's in kids or adults. The room kids have for junk is still small in relative terms. Thus, it's helpful for parents and guardians to teach and guide their children to use this room wisely in practical terms, so they can form good eating habits and have great health, while also enjoying their lives. As these children grow into teenagers, with the right knowledge and understanding acquired, they will adjust their choices to reflect recommended adult ratios as they get to further understand the value of their choices on their health. Children who obtain success in this area, generally tend to reflect the choices of their parents/guardians. For this reason, it is very important to model good choices at home, in order to promote your children's confidence in their abilities to make their personal good choices.

Generally, children are able to make good decisions, including food-related decisions, when they understand its value to them. If you are a parent or guardian, it's important you make time to help your children now, so you can equip them with a great foundation to be successful in their future. Involve them in making choices when you go to the grocery store, establish the importance of why certain foods will only make it to your pantry occasionally, and why certain foods would always be on your grocery list every time, in relating to boosting the body's immune health.

During my undergraduate years in biology, I worked occasionally as an intern in my dad's clinic in Ghana, where I personally witnessed certain men's health issues such as prostate-related conditions, as well as certain gynecological issues, respiratory issues, and lots of other health-related issues, resolve from trying some of these simple plant foods. My dad was always a firm believer in quality and bought these teas from large farms in Europe, solely dedicated to growing some of these herbs. These farms had measures in place to ensure good quality of their produce.

It is no wonder in my time of personal crisis as I described earlier, my mind was able to reconnect to some of these success stories, as I embarked on my own personal success journey. I am grateful to God that He made it happen for me, and allowed me to live, so I could tell my story and, hopefully, help prevent you from going through what I had to go through. I drink some of these teas occasionally when I am unable to find recipes that I can include them in, or sometimes simply for the unique flavor, while also obtaining their health benefits. The potential benefits of plant foods to our health is worth exploring. Certain herbal teas, right from the heart of your kitchen can make a difference in your health.

Occasionally, I choose a period within a month, in about every 4-6 months, during which I personally select a food-based regimen, and which can include teas with potential immune health-boosting capabilities. This period can be anywhere between 1-3 weeks within the designated month, depending on the foods I choose to target, how I feel, or simply, what I choose to do. During this period, I simply increase my frequency of consumption of the chosen food or group of foods, with an aim of increasing the concentration of their health-beneficial substances (health-beneficial bioactive compounds), within my body. While at this goal, I also keep my *concept of moderation* at heart, while *"tactfully"* and *"purposefully"* increasing the frequency of consumption of my chosen food(s). I keep this very simple, and many times, my increase in frequency is as basic as setting a daily consumption goal during the given period, as against maybe, a few times in a week per my normal routine.

Sometimes, my selection an herbal tea, or a specific food. My choice depends on what I decide to focus on that month as pertaining to my health, with immune health-boosting foods, typically at the center of my focused selections. In those months, should I choose to include any herbal foods in the form of teas, I like to drink those herbal teas, on an empty stomach, first thing in the morning, about 10-20 minutes before I eat my breakfast. I've found this timing to empower absorption and effectiveness, and I can tell by how I feel at the end of those months. I base this personal regimen on the concepts I discussed in Chapter 8. I have derived many personal everyday regimens from some of the discussed concepts. Please believe me when I tell you I wholeheartedly trust you can also derive many personal benefits based on an understanding of some of these concepts.

Generally, it is almost impossible to absolutely prevent potentially dangerous substances from entering your body, however hard you may try to prevent their entrance. For this reason, ways to seamlessly enhance your health by boosting its immune capabilities from within, is invaluable. Like I discussed in Chapter 8, sometimes passive ways, as from the air we breathe, as well as from many other avenues we may not even have control over, could create chances for some of these potentially dangerous substances to enter the body. Given all these, a major strategic action you can take is to consciously provide your body with reasonable amounts of antioxidants, anti-inflammatories, and other potential immune health boosters through the foods you eat. Doing this can help your body to take good care of its internal environment, which can be in the form of cleaning out some unintended potential toxins that might make their way into the body, or putting out unnecessary "fires" that could start, as in the case of the initial formation of diseased tissues (could include potential tumor cells). Yes, you can empower your body to perform its essential functions effectively.

In addition to some of my recommended kitchen must-haves and many other foods out there you can explore with tips from your favorite recipe books, good quality herbal teas can help you to achieve the objective of boosting your immune health. Outside of the 1-3 weeks about every 4-6 months I deliberately set aside to boost my immune health, I drink some of these teas occasionally when I feel like, to further support my health goals. Keep in mind your weight when drinking some of these teas. I am petite, and many times, a simple one teaspoon of loose herbal tea in one cup of hot water is a low dose, sufficient to take care of my needs. "Listen" to your body's needs, start with low doses; and read labels and instructions for guidance.

From general observation, I have found that for an individual with average weight, it is easy to obtain benefits from a light flavor of any tea by using 1 to 1.5 teaspoons of loose leaves to an 8-ounce cup of hot water. To obtain a medium to strong flavor, an average of 2-3 teaspoons to the 8-ounce cup seems to do the trick. Keep in mind the prevention of potential overconsumption of higher quantities, when exploring tea forms of herbs, most especially in loose herbal forms. Consumption in food-safe quantities is the ideal, and best way.

"Listen" to your body, and it will tell you what works best for you. Keep in mind the importance of apportioning foods to align with your body weight requirements and health goals. Always start slow, do not go overboard. Even a good thing can be harmful to you when consumed in excesses. Always drink in normal food quantities to reap the best benefits for your health, and read labels as in other foods, to help with safe levels of consumption. These are helpful tips, worth noting, when it comes to drinking health-beneficial teas

An ability to obtain essential benefits from certain herbal teas (as from their high antioxidant contents) while concurrently refraining from consuming artificial sweeteners or excessive sugars is important. This approach to drinking herbal teas can give you an upper hand in regulating dietary sugar intake, in comparison to most of the juices on the market. By the way, keep in mind a word of caution when buying juices; always read labels and stay attentive to all contained ingredients, even when it says 100% juice on the label. Being able to maintain good control over your weight management goals can many times tie into this tip, in addition to the many others described. Most herbal teas are best enjoyed without milk. There are a few though that lend themselves easily to the addition of milk, such as green tea (benefits of milk in green tea further discussed under green tea). Some also taste great with honey. When I go for honey, I prefer the organic unfiltered form, as I reap the most benefits from this form. Read labels, make your preferred picks.

For fans of juicing, the concept of absorption of herbal tea in the digestive tract can be compared to that of the absorption of juices in the digestive tract, especially if you drink a few minutes before meals, when the stomach is not as full. Like juices, herbal teas can also be enjoyed at any time between meals, as desired. I am personally not a fan of the concept of juicing only, as I also accord high importance to the place of fiber from fruits and vegetables in our diet. The juices from our fruits and vegetables have been shown to absorb just as well in the digestive tract when eaten with their fiber components. However, herbal teas after preparation, present themselves naturally without fiber from the plant, and these can be well absorbed by the body also, giving you the chance to consume your fiber from your fruit. It's absolutely alright to enjoy freshly squeezed juices. As a matter of fact, I do that sometimes, and I obtain benefits from them as well. The key application here is the *concept of balance*: Be careful not to resort to juicing only, without consuming enough fiber in your diet daily.

Keep in mind the importance of maintaining a variety of healthy eating styles and reaping total benefits when it comes to eating right and maintaining a healthy lifestyle. Personally, when I set aside those occasional 1-3 weeks out of about every 4-6 months, to focus on empowering my body with "health-full" foods like I mentioned earlier, I do this deliberately with a highly focused goal of increasing the concentration of their health-beneficial bioactive substances within my body during those periods. Simple consumption of these foods does the trick for me, as I believe I give my body a "kick" in immune health-strengthening capabilities. Throughout my day, every day in those designated weeks whenever I choose to include teas in my regimen, I make sure to also enjoy the fiber from my fruits and vegetables like I normally do. Sufficient daily fiber intake is a very essential component of a healthy diet, as discussed in Chapter 3. Consider trying this concept of drinking teas in various ways, and find what works best for you.

When trying teas for the first time, exercise any precautions that may be necessary as you'd normally do when starting any new foods or regimen. Consult with your primary care physician, most especially if taking any prescribed medications, and of course, look out for any signs of allergic reactions.

I've highlighted these few teas here, although there are tons of them. I do this because these selected teas I discuss are common and can bring a wealth of benefits to your immune health.

Green Tea

This is one of the most common teas that can be found in most kitchens, but usually often underestimated. Green tea is known to be one of the most common household teas to have the highest concentration of flavonoids. These flavonoids give green tea a very high antioxidant property. Among others, various catechins including epigallocatechin gallate (EGCG), are the major bioactive compounds, or flavonoids, that give green tea its benefits to health.[1] If you are careful with not going overboard with caffeine like I am (remember the *concept of moderation* in avoiding excesses), it would interest you to know that when compared with fresh tea leaves, black tea, and oolong teas, green tea has a relatively lower content of caffeine, with only fresh tea leaves among the group of four, being lower than green tea in caffeine content.[2] Of high significance also, is the fact that these health-beneficial catechins are highest in green tea when comparing all four.[3] Be aware that these catechins are highest in the normal caffeinated forms of these teas.

Catechin extracts from green tea have been shown to have antioxidant, anticancer, and heart-related (cardiovascular) disease prevention properties.[4] The strong antioxidant and anti-inflammatory effects of EGCG extracts from green tea have been demonstrated to be effective in certain cells in the eyes (human corneal epithelial cells), with a potential of having healing (therapeutic) properties in ocular inflammatory conditions, as in dry eye.[5] There are tons of studies that support the antioxidant and anti-inflammatory properties shown by green tea.

Catechins have been shown to have protective (neuroprotective) effects against the destruction of nerve cells (oxidative damage and degeneration) in patients with Parkinson's disease who may also be receiving treatment.[6] Currently, no cure has been found for Parkinson's disease, but a lot is known about its progression, in how it negatively affects neurons, which are nerve cells in the nervous system (inclusive of the brain and the spinal cord) of the body. This negative effect causes a destruction of these neurons and stimulates many symptoms, that come along with the deterioration. To further complicate this condition, certain medications that currently help to lessen the symptoms such as levodopa (a widely used one), also come along with their own negative effects.

When taken for Parkinson's, the medication levodopa turns to dopamine within the body. Dopamine is a substance, naturally produced in the brain, that helps with the transmission of information, enabling communication between nerve cells, within the nervous system of the body. Normally, the body produces amounts needed for its function. However, in people with Parkinson's disease, this chemical substance (dopamine), is known to be produced at relatively low levels in the brain. This is the reason they take the medication levodopa, to help boost availability of the substance dopamine, within the body. On the flip side, although widely known for its effectiveness in handling disease-related symptoms, over time, when taken for lengthy periods, levodopa typically begins to lose its effectiveness. The potential loss of effectiveness of this otherwise great medication is often attributed to methylation of the levodopa. Not to go into details, the methylation of this medication is a chemical process levodopa undergoes over time within the body, that causes changes to its chemical structure, and hence, its effectiveness.

I explained this to give you a broad overview of what people with Parkinson's sometimes have to deal with, especially if the medication that was helping with managing their symptoms begins to take a downward spiral from doing its job. It is of much significance to state that catechins, specifically, EGCG, have been shown to be effective also in preventing this methylation of levodopa, in addition to its neuroprotective benefits.[7] This can thus help to keep the levodopa effective for longer and has a great potential of benefiting people being treated for Parkinson's disease. A simple cup of green tea can make a wealth of difference when it makes its way into the body. Go for it!

The antioxidant properties exhibited by these catechins are able to prevent oxidation of bad cholesterol as from the discussions in Chapter 10, while increasing the levels of good cholesterol. Based on the understanding you obtained from discussions from Chapter 10 of how this simple process can help curb heart disease, do you see how this simple food can help make a difference in the health of your heart? Of equally great significance is the potential cancer preventive effects[8] shown by flavonoids from green tea. The strong antioxidant effects shown by this amazing tea should not be underestimated.

Consider going for that cup of green tea. If you're concerned about the taste, keep in mind it's as a result of some of the health-beneficial flavonoid components from this tea. One thing I can tell you both from my personal experience and from scientific studies is that it is possible to train your tongue to get used to various flavors and tastes. The concept is the same as it relates to training your tongue to get used to "junk". By that same standard, you can practice training your tongue for some healthy picks, and believe me, it gets used to it over time. Your willingness to try great foods and regimens is key to achieving great immune health.

This is one of my favorite statements that keep me challenged, even in pursuit of my health goals: "where there is a will, there's always a way". Does this resonate with you as well? Your health is your most valuable asset, and it is worth making every effort necessary to take good care of it.

As a health professional, having seen so much, I can confidently tell you that when compared to the high cost of dealing with a debilitating health condition, the little things you can do to empower your body to stay in shape is trivial. Most especially when this comparison is associated with the need to train your taste buds to align with your health goals. With this understanding in mind, I train myself and my family to go for health-beneficial foods, including occasional green tea, given the enormous potential benefits these can bring to the body. I believe you can do the same if you are willing to consider trying.

Thankfully, in contrast to much speculation about the odds of drinking milk with your green teas, studies have shown that drinking green tea while also consuming dairy products, helps to maintain the green tea's bioactive (polyphenol) substance's integrity, as well as its antioxidant activity, during digestion.[9] This is great, as it can help with occasionally considering some green tea "sides" along with our meals, whether breakfast, lunches, or dinners. This provides a lot of room for creativity, whenever we choose to consume green teas.

In exploring green teas, like all other foods, keep quality at heart when making purchases, as well as all other precautions that pertain to foods, including those discussed throughout the book.

Mint

I have found it necessary to talk about mint broadly, as it tends to be a very common term. It is used largely and informally by most people in reference to plants that have the "minty" smell. Generally, these plants with the "minty" smell belong to the genus, *Mentha*, comprising of various plant species (about 15-20), with the most common being the peppermint (*Mentha piperita*) and spearmint (*Mentha spicata*). Keep in mind that technically and scientifically, the mint group of plants consist of plants from the family Lamiaceae, as I mentioned at the beginning of the chapter.

For the purpose of discussing the mint plant, keep Mentha in mind. Please also use the "minty" aroma as a guide, while also picturing your spearmint and peppermint as samples from this wide species of plants. Mint plants are common globally, with certain species being prevalent in certain regions, as with Spearmint in Europe and Asia, although it's widespread in many other regions. Most mint plants grow in wet environmental conditions and soils, although they are able to grow under a wide variety of conditions. This must be one reason why mint plants are widespread globally and are found in various geographical regions.

The robust "minty" flavor from mint plants is from the substance, menthol. This substance has many uses and is in high demand. It is used as a component in the production of many over the counter products, as in many inhalants for the common cold and nasal congestion. It is artificially produced in many industries to help meet its high demand. Like the discussion of thymol, menthol helps to further explain how research studies on plants help in studying the chemical structures of certain beneficial compounds which are then sometimes manufactured synthetically to help meet demand for larger quantities. I am saying this to support the fact that if you can obtain certain benefits from plants by eating them or using them in safe forms, by all means, consider taking advantage of them.

Mint has versatile uses in the culinary world, like many of its counterparts in the Lamiaceae family. It has a robust, unique flavor which it can contribute to enhancing many dishes. Whether in a fruit salad dessert or a drink, mint can bring that extra enrichment you need. Mint can also add extra flavor to your meats such as fish or lamb. For cooking, spearmint is the most commonly used.

Mint tea is one of my favorites. I particularly enjoy its flavor. The taste of mint teas can easily be heightened with lemons and honey to make some awesome drinks. You and your loved ones can consider exploring various recipes of mint drinks at home together, enjoy them, and even use them as substitutes for sodas. These can come in handy most especially during the winter days, to help curb the frequency of, as well as alleviate common respiratory congestions. Some of these robust-flavored drinks like mint can get even bolder in taste when ginger is thrown into mixes containing them. When you want to spice things up a little more, ginger can help you go up a notch higher not only in taste but also in immune health-boosting capabilities. These tips will provide a broad idea of some of the strategies you can explore while trying to include mint in your diet. I hope you find some of them helpful when you choose to make tweaks to some of your favorite recipes, with an aim of creating a wider variety of your preferred dishes, drinks, or desserts.

In the grocery store, mint can be bought in potted plant packaging or other fresh forms, as well as in tea packages. These tend to be the most popular forms, as most people enjoy mint fresh or in tea. Although there are dried forms of mint mostly found in the spice aisles, the best flavor is obtained from fresh mint. If you are like me, you may prefer to choose the tea packaging as well whenever possible, or find yourself with a choice over mint spices. I think I get the most robust flavors from the teas and fresh forms, and I believe you may find the same as well.

There are also essential oils made from the mint plant, available on the market. Aromatherapy lovers enjoy benefits from the mint plant. The various forms of mint follow the same convention when buying and storing, as those described for others in the family like rosemary and thyme. As in any other foods or products, keep quality at heart when buying mint in any form.

Why Mint?

Mint is popularly known for its aroma and flavor. It is no wonder its use is prevalent in aromatherapy. It's unique aroma also makes it popular in the treatment of the common cold and obtaining relief from respiratory discomforts of such nature. Mint has also been predominant in its beneficial use for gastrointestinal discomforts, such as indigestion and nausea. Mint has been shown to have protective effects on the lining of the stomach, even in situations of stomach ulcers that are caused by certain medications (drug-induced gastric ulcer)[1], as in what possibly results from the long-term use of drugs like ibuprofen.

Some of the most widely used species of mint studied is the peppermint, and it has been found to have properties that prevent unwanted oxidation (antioxidant), "fight" against viruses (antiviral), "fight" against bacteria (antibacterial), allergic reaction-minimizing or "fighting" (antiallergenic), and "tumor-fighting" (antitumor) effects.[2]

Menthol, a major bioactive substance found in the mint plant and which gives the plant its unique "minty" flavor, has actually been isolated and found to have "bacteria-fighting" properties[3], giving meaning to its effectiveness in the treatment of a sore throat and minor throat irritations. In this study, it was shown to be effective against some common bacteria (some of which are responsible for some common infections), such as *Streptococcus mutans*, *Staphylococcus aureus*, and the common yeast, *Candida albicans*, just to mention a few. Some of these bacteria are very common in everyday encounters. For example, *Candida albicans* is notable as a cause of the common yeast infection, as mentioned in an earlier discussion. *Staphylococcus aureus* is a prevalent skin bacterium, also widespread in the cause of many minor skin infections.

A cup of peppermint tea from your kitchen has a potential to do wonders for your body, and can act to prevent the multiplication of certain bacteria to levels that are high enough to probably cause an infection. In other words, you may be able to stop some bacterial actions right in their tracks even when you are not aware, from your simple consumption of mint. It is no wonder lots of brands of mouthwash utilize the properties of menthol and thymol in enhancing their "bacteria-fighting" effects.

Flavonoids, including rosmarinic acid, of which you are familiar by now from previous discussions, and others like isorhoifolin (shown to have the most potent effect in mint's bioactive properties), isolated from the peppermint plant, have been noted to have an ability to inhibit the release of histamine.[4] The release of histamine is a very important step, necessary especially to result in a runny nose in people who typically have a runny nose stimulated by allergens (allergic rhinitis) such as pollen. You may be familiar with lots of over the counter antihistamines that help to alleviate these symptoms many times. People who suffer from this condition may be able to obtain relief from trying peppermint if they do not have any allergies to it as well.

Mint's decongestant property[5], along with its calming effect, are attributes that make it versatile in its use in aromatherapy. For instance, it has been renowned to stimulate a calming effect in people experiencing fatigue and its potentially associated headaches. Improved lung function and exercise capacities have been obtained by the use of mint essential oils in a study using athletes as study participants.[6] Results from this study actually have a recommendation for further studies in this area. This could potentially lead to many possible uses of mint in the near future, most especially as an aid to boosting response to conventional treatments of certain conditions.

The capability of mint in inhibiting the growth of certain tumor cells (antitumor property), as well as its potential property as an antioxidant[7] in preventing the oxidation and the removal of oxidizing agents from the body that could be potentially harmful to it, is very significant. This is because the more of foods that have an ability to rid the body of free radicals that we consume, the better it is for our health (see Chapter 8). An application of this concept is very necessary for us in strengthening our bodies and getting the body into a mode that can potentially empower its disease-prevention capabilities.

The list goes on, even in the use of mint in cosmetics. For people battling a condition that causes patches of baldness known as alopecia, it may be worth the mention that peppermint oil extract containing 3% peppermint, has been shown to promote hair growth in just about 4 weeks without showing signs of toxicity.[8] This is significant, as most drugs used for treating this condition have shown some toxic effects as well.

Enjoying a variety of foods from the mint family, including the mint plant itself, can be very helpful in boosting our immune health. Whatever your preferences are, I am glad this family of plants affords the convenience of consuming and using them in a variety of ways so we can tailor choices to our particular needs and taste. Whether you'd love to simply drink teas made from mint, season your meats with it, or even include it in your dessert recipes, there is a wide range of options to choose from. By all means, consider making your picks from the wide variety of available recipes, and keep them handy by adding the forms of mint you'd need to your list of kitchen must-haves.

Like any of the other foods discussed, some people may be allergic to mint, and it's important to look out for any potential allergies, especially if trying these for the first time. The *concept of moderation* in the sense of consuming in normal food quantities is highly recommended in the consumption of mint, as in any other foods. Remember, even the best of foods when over-eaten, can potentially lead to a negative consequence. I hope you'll take advantage of the benefits that the mint plant and members of its family of plants can potentially bring to your health.

CHAPTER TWENTY-TWO

Superfoods In Review

Health-beneficial substances in various foods tend
to have their unique approaches in carrying out
their health-beneficial functions. Eat a variety!

In recent years, the concept of superfoods has been refer-
enced by a lot of experts in the food industry. Superfoods
are, simply put, foods that have been categorized as having
a rich nutritional content, particularly of great benefit to our
health. These benefits are derived from many bioactive compounds contained in these foods that can potentially provide
many benefits to the body. In this chapter, I discuss superfoods
in the light of their nutrient-rich constituents. Depending on
what your focus is in searching or categorizing, you can find a
wide variety of foods that can be placed in any one category.
And yes indeed, many foods will fall into any single category
you choose to create. From spinach to salmon, and beans, many
foods can meet this criterion of "nutrient-rich" based on what
nutrients you choose to base your focus/categorization on.

These superfoods are named because they tend to have relatively higher quantities of certain health beneficial bioactive substances in comparison to many others, as in some of those discussed. I say this to say that there is a wide range of "healthfull" superfoods, and it's important to find your preferences based on your particular needs, most especially if there are some you do not particularly care for. With that said, continue to keep in mind though, that the tongue can be trained, and you can choose to do that, especially for the benefit of your health if you need to. Your needs can be seasonal. Based on the *concepts of moderation and balance* discussed, strategically eating a wide variety of health-beneficial foods can potentially give you the best results when it comes to boosting your immune health.

I selectively discuss a few outstanding beneficial bioactive compounds, with pointers to some popular foods that contain some of these. In the discussions, I use an approach that will help you to mentally "visualize" how some of these special compounds span across some basic foods, as well as the wide variety available for you to choose from. The more of these you eat, the more advantage you give to your body in boosting its immune health. You can consider using some of these foods to your health's advantage.

The goal of this chapter is to challenge you to form a mental picture and have an even greater understanding of your food choices and how these choices can potentially impact your health. I hope this stirs your interest in beginning to analyze the foods you eat so you can empower your health mentally, emotionally, and physically, for a better lifestyle and happier you.

The great attributes of some these wonderful bioactive substances, or rich nutrients, as I simply put them, is that they afford these superfoods the benefits that place them in the category of certain superfoods. Most importantly, these amazing "health-full" nutrients tend to be available in a wide variety of foods, in varying quantities. Knowledge of some of these foods and an idea of the average quantities of these rich nutrients contained in them will be helpful to you as you make your preferred choices of health-boosting foods. I also use this approach of discussing superfoods in terms of nutrients because, in as much as eating a variety is important, I understand there are times when someone may absolutely not like a particular immune health-boosting food for certain reasons, or even be allergic to some of these foods. However, I do believe even under these circumstances, it is possible to find alternate immune health-boosting foods of your preference that could still get the job done.

Personal challenges should not stop anyone from obtaining corresponding health-boosting nutrients from other foods when possible. There are wide varieties of foods that contain any particular health-beneficial substance. Surely, you and your loved ones can find what works best for you. There are many tips for preparing some of these nutrient-rich foods in various ways that can help you to enjoy them while on your journey to empowering your health. Of particular importance to me is the knowledge this will provide in helping you to boost your immune health, with an accompanying boost to your overall health.

Kaempferol

You may be wondering, what is Kaempferol? This gets even better, as it has many other names including Kaempherol, Robigenin, Trifolitin[1], just to mention a few. As strange as it sounds, this is a potent health-beneficial compound found prevalently in a variety of plants, and certain foods made from plants. This amazing plant compound (or flavonoid) has potent antioxidant properties that have earned it a place in ongoing research studies for the prevention and reduction of risks in the occurrence of many diseases, inclusive of cancers.

Kaempferol, in its action as an antioxidant, is able to decrease oxidative stress. This mode of action makes it worth discussing, as it is a potent immune health booster, in alignment with the discussion in Chapter 3, with regards to the role of antioxidants in boosting immune health. Of great significance is the fact that Kaempferol is naturally occurring in varying quantities in a wide variety of plant foods, thus leaving room for many of us to easily make our preferred picks. Some of the most common foods that contain kaempferol include broccoli, cabbage, kale, green beans, onions, green tea, lettuce, squash, tomatoes, grapes, spinach, and much more.

I believe that although health-beneficial results have been obtained in studies using kaempferol, it has not been given as much extensive attention and publicity. Kaempferol can inhibit the growth of certain cancer cells, while also causing them to destroy themselves.[2] Not only can it do these in cancer cells, but it also appears to have a protective function of normal cells.[3] This is in sharp contrast to many cancer treatments that exert destructive effects on normal cells in their attempt to destroy cancerous tissue. This has been a great concern in the medical community as more research continues in the quest of finding cures for this deadly disease. Who knows, this could possibly be one of the leads to better treatments for certain cancer patients, as studies strive to find most potent forms of extraction, and quantities that are able to exert the best effects. Until then, one of the greatest benefits you can give to your body is in the consumption of foods that are rich in kaempferol.

It's amazing to come across foods that can be of help in empowering the body to fight any such cell(s) or growth that may potentially raise its head to bring the body down, as in cancer cells. It is important to point out that Kaempferol can obstruct a number of inflammatory processes[4], giving it an anti-inflammatory property. Kaempferol can increase blood sugar (glucose) uptake as well as positively influence certain metabolic disorders associated with obesity and aging.[5] It also has an ability to enhance the production and function of insulin in the body, very important in preventing diabetes. In this capacity, kaempferol can improve peripheral insulin sensitivity and protect certain cells in the pancreas responsible for storage and release of insulin (beta cells), giving it a natural anti-diabetic property.[6]

The anti-inflammatory property of kaempferol has been shown to work well against nervous system-related inflammation processes (neuroinflammatory processes)[7], giving it a favorable pick as having neuroprotective properties. Remember, when you think of neuroprotective properties, think about the nervous system which can include brain health-boosting capabilities, as we have seen previously in the various discussions of certain brain conditions, as in Parkinson's disease. Furthermore, certain pathways of bone metabolism disorders have been shown to be effectively disrupted by the action of kaempferol[8], giving it a positive look hopefully in the future as well, in the search for certain bone disorder treatments like osteoporosis.

Certain female disorders have responded favorably to the actions of kaempferol. It has shown to effectively inhibit the growth and multiplication of certain uterine fibroid cells.[9] A caution on its ability to possibly inhibit fertility[10] should also be noted. This can be of concern if being consumed outside of normal food quantity amounts. This further substantiates the *concept of variety and moderation* in getting best results from foods, widely discussed throughout the book. In addition to having many other outstanding properties, Kaempferol is a major plant compound that contributes to giving broccoli, cabbage, and most cruciferous vegetables (plants in the cabbage family), their cancer-fighting capabilities.

Kaempferol has been known to have many medicinal (pharmacological) properties, inclusive of antioxidant, anti-inflammatory, and anti-cancer.[11] I could continue to elaborate on many other properties that this amazing flavonoid has, but I believe the few I have mentioned so far are more than enough to help you form a mental picture of the amazing benefits you could potentially obtain from including kaempferol-rich foods in your diet.

This great nutrient is found in lots of plant foods, as from the examples given. Increasing your consumption of plant foods, most especially in ways that are strategic enough to accommodate a wide variety can help to cover a lot of bases in enhancing your health. I hope that the next time you fill your dinner plate, you have been challenged well enough to ensure that at least half of your plate is covered with your vegetables and fruits. Additionally, whenever you think of snacking, I hope you think of plant foods. Most importantly, be sure to include plants that contain the flavonoid kaempferol in your diet, to help enhance your health.

Luteolin

Luteolin is another flavonoid, that has a potential to contribute immensely to boosting your immune health. It is another compound found in a wide variety of plant foods, thereby, also contributing to the importance of the *concept of eating a wide variety* of foods, most especially plant foods. Luteolin can be found in citrus plants, some leaves, certain aromatic flowering plants, and many others. Thus, certain common foods that contain luteolin include navel oranges, carrots, olive oil, green pepper, celery, broccoli, parsley, basil, thyme, peppermint, rosemary, and oregano.[1]

I hope you see a trend in the family Lamiaceae (the Mint Family), beautifully represented, as well as certain foods that are known to be potential providers of certain other flavonoids, as in broccoli. This trend helps to even further solidify the fact that your little counts and the little you may do could go a long way and will certainly be better than doing nothing. The value of your choices adds up over time. The few sticks of carrots you may nibble on as snacks, or even substitute for a side of fries, could potentially add up to what you do overall at the end of the day or week, in contributing to boosting your immune health.

Additionally, finding plant foods you prefer, and eating those in good quantities can potentially go a long way to enhance the state of your health. This should stir you into eating a good amount of vegetables, and throwing in some basil, thyme, rosemary, etc. to spice up your cooking and your health. Luteolin is worth paying attention to, because like many of our flavonoids, it has antioxidant, anti-inflammatory, and anti-tumor properties.

Tumor cells including cancer cells have "strategic" ways of arming themselves to thrive, grow, and invade the environment within which they begin to flourish. For this reason, many times, different approaches and treatments are utilized by teams of specialists, when treating patients dealing with such tumor growth challenges, with hopes of landing on a method that best treats a situation.

Having been in the medical field for so long, I can tell you that one size does not always fit all. This is a concept I have consistently discussed, and I continue to emphasize. For this same reason, you'll also realize that many flavonoids in their "fight" against let's say some bacteria, or even a tumor growth, tend to use strategies that are unique to them. Hence, the wider the range of flavonoids we incorporate into our food choices, the better we are at arming our bodies, by putting in place a wide range of nutritionally rich defenses that can boost our immune health and our overall state of health. This, in turn, will put the body in a position of strength to better "fight" pathogens, unwanted growth, or potentially harmful substances that may attempt to "overpower" it.

I say this to state that luteolin is armed with its own unique ability to defend the body, that earns it the ability to make its way to the list of flavonoids with antioxidant, anti-inflammatory and anti-tumor properties. Without going into extensive detail with regards to how luteolin does this, let me mention that luteolin has been shown to inhibit the growth of human prostate tumor cells[2] via its own unique defense mechanism in the process. It's able to do this effectively by working to prevent the effective formation of new blood vessels responsible for this growth by negatively impacting the inner lining[3] of such blood vessels. The growth and ability of these tumor cells to thrive is heavily dependent on the effective formation and functioning of the new blood vessels that continually form around them, and which also arm them with what they need to grow. Hence, interfering with the proper functioning of the blood vessels that nourish such tumors would in turn affect the ability of their corresponding tumors to thrive.

Luteolin's ability to interfere with the effective growth and multiplication of such blood vessels that surround human prostate tumor cells is worth paying attention to. It gets even better. Luteolin can disrupt the migration and invasion of certain tumor cells of the brain, usually cancerous, known as glioblastoma cells.[4] These glioblastomas typically tend to be cancerous and are highly invasive, armed with a strong ability to grow rapidly, because they can make their own blood supply and propagate themselves with great aggression.

Luteolin has strong anti-cancer properties exhibited in its multiple strategies, such as having an ability to prevent cellular growth/multiplication of these cancer cells (inhibition of cell proliferation), disrupting the formation of new blood vessels (angiogenesis) in these cells, interfering with these cancer cells' ability to invade healthy tissue (metastasis), and the ability to induce self-destruction in these cancer cells (apoptosis).[5] Various studies have shown these properties of luteolin, making it one worth paying attention to. Luteolin also has the capability of fighting against certain allergies (anti-allergenic properties).[6] All these support the fact that eating a variety of foods rich in luteolin can boost the body's immune health.

Just to cite a simple but easy potential benefit that can be obtained from Luteolin as pertaining to its antioxidant properties, let me use an illustration of diabetic neuropathy. This is a potential complication in diabetics who are unable to successfully manage their blood sugars. This condition typically results in nerve damage usually with effects experienced in the legs, feet, and over time, other parts of the body in certain diabetics who struggle with effective control of their blood sugar. This condition can cause a lot of pain in the affected body parts, for people who suffer from it. It's important to state that the antioxidant and neuroprotective effects of luteolin have been shown to be potentially beneficial to improving diabetes-related neuropathy[7], which typically causes problems in sensory and motor functions of individuals who suffer from this condition. This can potentially lead to beneficial insights in this area, as pertaining to diabetic care in the future. Until then, why not obtain your share of this great flavonoid from the foods you eat, in this season of your life? Your little strides can go a long way. Don't underestimate them.

Luteolin has shown potential benefits to the heart, in its ability to protect heart cells (having cardioprotective abilities)[8] as well. Not only in protecting, but luteolin also has a capability to improve the heart cell's capacity to contract and function in pumping and circulating blood within the body, even after an injury to the heart tissue.[9] Of great benefit to the immune system is the anti-inflammatory property of luteolin. This has been shown in various studies, including a study on a common organ-specific autoimmune disease known as Hashimoto's thyroiditis. Recall that in autoimmune diseases, the body turns against its own tissues, sees them as foreign, begins to attack, and in many cases, destroys those tissues. In Hashimoto's thyroiditis, the attack is against the thyroid, and those affected many times in addition to other symptoms, tend to show a swelling of their thyroid around their neck region. In displaying its benefits in alleviating this disease, luteolin exerts an influence by suppressing the immune response (immunosuppressant effect)[10] within the body. It does this by tactically acting on various steps of the inflammatory process that leads to the cause of the disease. We also see its anti-inflammatory property shown in various other functions, as in luteolin's cardioprotective and neuroprotective properties, mentioned earlier.

We see some of the various health benefits that can be obtained from luteolin, simply by eating a wide variety of plant foods that are rich in it. Consider eating luteolin-rich foods while research continues to unearth even more health benefits that would hopefully impact the future of finding cures for certain diseases. I hope all this helps you to visualize the fact that you can impact your health by including a wide variety of plant foods in your food choices. Be innovative and go for health benefits while you enjoy your foods, keeping luteolin-containing foods in mind.

Myricetin

Myricetin is a flavonoid with great potential health benefits. It can be commonly found in a wide range of plant foods. In the food industry, especially where benefits of food to the body are explored (nutraceuticals), this is widely known because of its worth. Antioxidant, anti-cancer, antidiabetic and anti-inflammatory properties[1], to name a few, have been attributed to myricetin. Lots of studies tend to focus on a cluster of several flavonoids at a time, with myricetin typically studied alongside others, as well as in comparison to others.

The antioxidant potential of myricetin has been shown to be much stronger than that of Vitamin E, even 28 times more potent in speed when reacting with certain free radicals.[2] One way of picturing some of these flavonoids is in their variety of colors and sources. Each of these unique fruits and vegetables bring something special to our health from their rich components. Worth noting is the fact that each of these flavonoids and health-beneficial substances found in various foods tend to have their unique approaches in exhibiting or carrying out their health-beneficial functions. For example, even though myricetin and, let's say, cinnamon may both contribute to decreasing type 2 diabetes risks, each has a peculiar way of effecting this property as a potential antidiabetic. For this reason, it is needful to say again that the *concept of eating a wide variety* of healthful foods is very necessary for arming your body with defenses to better carry out its functions within your immune system.

Some of the common foods that are rich in myricetin include onions (particularly the red), grapes, walnuts, berries (blueberries, cranberries, and especially blackberries), and much more. Red wine has myricetin also, though many of us like myself choose to steer away from it because of the alcoholic content. Particularly worth noting is grapes' rich content in a wide range of health-beneficial flavonoids, inclusive of myricetin, kaemp-ferol, and quercetin among others. I love to snack on them to-gether with carrots, a delicious combination for snack you can consider trying.

Myricetin has been shown to have protective capabilities against obesity and insulin resistance that are caused by diet.[3] In this study noted and various others, we see a display of myrice-tin in its ability to decrease blood glucose levels, regulate the metabolism of fat (lipid), and mount a protective attack against high-fat-diet-induced oxidative stress[4], in achieving the results obtained. These are further reflective of antidiabetic and antiox-idant properties of Myricetin among others mentioned.

With such potency exhibited, inclusive of its anti-inflamma-tory properties shown from various studies, it is no wonder that still other studies have shown its anti-cancer capabilities as well. There are typically strong relationships between anti-inflamma-tory and antioxidant properties in flavonoids, and anti-cancer properties, as well as many other disease-fighting capabilities of substances. The more you pay attention to some of these special flavonoids and use them in boosting your immune health capa-bilities, the better the chances you may have at keeping diseases away from your body, most especially with a focus on those dis-eases with unknown causes.

Myricetin shows several properties that are of benefit to the central nervous system, and various studies have shown that this flavonoid may provide protection against diseases related to this system, as in Parkinson's and Alzheimer's.[5]

Myricetin has been shown to have a strong ability to induce the death of various cancer cells (apoptosis), including ovari-an cancer cells[6] by various mechanisms of action. Lung cancer cells have also shown an enhanced death effect with exposure to myricetin, while at the same time undergoing an exposure to radiation treatment.[7] The myricetin in this combination of the trial seems to enhance a better action of the radiation treatment in its "killing" of the lung cancer tumor cells. This shows that this flavonoid could potentially be used effectively in enhancing other treatments targeted at destroying certain cancerous cells in the future.

I hope these highlights challenge you enough to consider taking this step toward including myricetin-rich foods in your diet, or even doing more if you are already in the habit.

Quercetin

Quercetin is another potent flavonoid, found in a wide variety of plant foods. Quercetin has been shown scientifically to have health-beneficial properties, inclusive of antioxidant, anticarcinogenic, anti-inflammatory and antiviral properties.[1]

Within the body, sometimes free radicals can cause a "snatching" of electrons from the lipids of cell membranes. This offsets the same destructive pathways as in those described earlier in how free radicals act in posing danger within the body when allowed to accumulate in large proportions. This can lead to cell damage and is termed lipid peroxidation, because it aims at the lipid in the cellular membrane. Quercetin has been shown to have an ability to weaken such lipid peroxidation activities[2], which is a real plus when it comes to dealing with free radicals and their potential negative effects within the body.

Quercetin has an ability to weaken the clumping together (aggregation) of blood platelets.[3] This is notable, as clumping of platelets in the blood is an essential step that typically leads to blood clot formation within the body. The clumping mechanism can easily take place in various functional systems or parts of the body, most commonly in the cardiac system, often traced in heart attacks, and many others. Many people with a potential of easily having blood clots form within their body by platelet clumping (aggregation) take various prescribed medications. The medications aim at interfering with, and weakening the process. As you can see, the capabilities of quercetin to interfere with these potentially dangerous processes may be particularly beneficial and could very well be the factors that give quercetin amazing potential benefits to the heart and the body's cholesterol management mechanisms.

One important reason for highlighting quercetin is its great potential in enhancing the health of the heart. Quercetin extract obtained from onion skin and given in a clinical study in amounts of 162mg/day to hypertensive patients was able to lower ambulatory blood pressure in some of the study participants.[4] This and many similar studies have shown a cardioprotective property of quercetin as relating to blood pressure management. Some participants and studies using different study factors have shown various other results. For example, a study looking at blood pressure after a meal, which was conducted on overweight to obese patients fed high fat and high carbohydrate diets, did not reveal a lowering effect on blood pressure when these study participants were given quercetin.[5] This study conducted by the same group of researchers who obtained the blood pressure-lowering effect earlier cited, indicate that like most other studies and foods, different factors could alter results.

In yet another study, all participants, also obese, showed a significant reduction in systolic blood pressure[6], which is the number on the top half of your blood pressure reading. Factors as in monitoring after the consumption of a high fat, high carbohydrate diet were not at play. There is a definite trend of potential cardioprotective benefits shown from many studies done on quercetin. To attain these benefits, try to consume quercetin in food quantities, while also maintaining other nutritionally beneficial heart healthy habits, as in consuming low amounts of "unhealthy fat" from diet and many others, discussed earlier.

Both quercetin and luteolin have been shown to reduce high blood cholesterol levels by various mechanisms, inclusive of preventing absorption of intestinal cholesterol.[7] It is no wonder that this flavonoid has been shown to have various benefits on the cardiovascular system. Most of these benefits, as in the potential of decreasing atherosclerosis, take advantage of quercetin's strong antioxidant and anti-inflammatory properties, while also using various mechanisms, as in the prevention of intestinal cholesterol absorption.

Quercetin's strong antiviral properties have been shown in various studies, including even an anti-influenza activity in a study. In this study, quercetin was able to inhibit influenza infection in the early stage by inhibiting entry of the H5N1 virus, thus the Influenza A virus.[8]

Many other benefits of quercetin have been shown to the body's health. Quercetin has been shown to have strong anti-cancer properties with various mechanisms of action that scientists continue to study. Quercetin has been noted to effectively work against various cancer cells, including prostate cancer cells[9] and inducing self-destruction (apoptosis) in a certain type of breast cancer cells (estrogen receptor positive)[10], to name a few. Studies indicate a simple consumption of quercetin, specifically from your fruits and vegetables, can provide protective effects from various forms of cancer.[11] What you eat matters, and again, by carefully aiming at eating health-beneficial foods, as in quercetin-rich foods, you may be able to give your body an edge to better protect and sustain itself.

Note that quercetin can be found in a wide variety of foods, including peppers, citrus fruits, apples (especially unpeeled), berries (blueberries, blackberries, etc.), dark cherries, tomatoes, grapes, onions especially red and yellow sweet, many seeds and nuts, green leafy vegetables (spinach, kale, etc.), cruciferous vegetables (broccoli, cabbage, etc.), and many more. I hope you see a pattern in colors and flavonoids here, and the necessity of eating a wide variety of fruits and vegetables.

For all these benefits and more, I hope you are considering enriching your diet with fruits and vegetables loaded with quercetin.

CHAPTER TWENTY-THREE

The True Superheroes

The "Little drops" matter and can make a
big difference in your long-term health.
Do not take them lightly, keep on adding!

Y ou may be wondering who or what these superheroes
are. Who doesn't want to know a superhero? I call
flavonoids the true superheroes. This is because I believe they save the day. You'll find out what they are and why
I say so, as you read on. In this chapter, I find it necessary to
discuss the subject of flavonoids, in close relation to my previous discussion on superfoods. This is because I find it helpful in
using the subject of flavonoids to further elaborate on some of
the nutrient-rich bioactive substances in plant foods, and some
of which I have discussed throughout the book. Some foods
have earned the title of "superfoods", because of their potential
benefits to the body.

Flavonoids are a class of plant-based compounds, or pig-
ments, and can be found in almost all fruits and vegetables in

multiple varieties and quantities. In a broad sense, flavonoids include over six thousand phenolic compounds.[1] Thank God for plants! They may be awkward-looking and sounding in terms of their names, but don't let flavonoids put you off from understanding them and using them to your advantage. Flavonoids can add a wealth of benefits to our health. I'm so glad we can eat them without needing to sound their names, most especially once we understand their value to our health.

Having read about kaempferol, luteolin, myricetin, quercetin, as well as others mentioned throughout the book, it is very important to me that you remember that these are very few of the many health-beneficial flavonoids available to us from plant foods. I chose to discuss these because of their value and how easy it is to obtain foods that contain them. In fact, from the over six thousand flavonoids identified by scientists like I stated, the ones I have mentioned and discussed are only a few from some of the major common ones. In addition to the value these can add to health and the relative ease of obtaining them from certain common foods, I chose to discuss the selected few so you would be able to relate to the amazing potential benefits fruits, and vegetables can bring to your personal health.

Generally, flavonoids typically tend to add color pigmentation to some of the foods that contain them, whether it's the green color of your spinach, or the red color of your grapes, and much more. Multiple flavonoids can, and usually tend to be present in any one particular plant food. This is very important, as the more you eat in terms of quantity, frequency, or variety, the higher the chances you have of getting good amounts of these rich flavonoids into your bloodstream. Flavonoids tend to be essential to boosting immune health, as most tend to have anti-inflammatory, antioxidant, anti-cancer, and even anti-bacterial and antiviral properties, as in some discussed.

From various scientific studies noted, we see some of their potential benefits to various body systems, inclusive of the digestive, nervous, cardiac, endocrine, and much more. Many times, these multiple combinations of flavonoids in various plant foods tend to further boost the potency of each other, leading to an increase in their potential benefit to our health. For this reason and others, being that they work in many ways, the more variety of plant foods you eat, the better the potential boost you can give to your immune health.

Keep in mind that when you eat, the food must go through various processes of digestion, and then finally have nutrients absorbed, making those nutrients available for use within the body. Now, this is where *"bioavailability"* comes into play. The bioavailability of the nutrients from the foods you eat, as in that from these flavonoids, is the amount of the flavonoid, that is successfully able to go through the process of digestion, get absorbed in the intestines, and then become available within the bloodstream, for use by the various cells, tissues, and organs of the body.

For many of the foods we eat, not all the potentially beneficial nutrients, including those from flavonoids, become available for use within the body. This is as a potential result of various probable "glitches" that sometimes interfere with food's total digestion, inclusive of absorption within the body. In addition to discussing the importance of combining foods in various ways that enhance better digestion and absorption (be sure to check out some of the previously discussed tips), I find it necessary to emphasize that some of these flavonoids complement each other in terms of enhancing each other's benefits to the body. Thus, further supporting the importance of eating a wide variety of foods with different flavonoids. Furthermore, many of these flavonoids have different ways of working within the body, and these different ways of action can come together to enhance the overall action of a benefit within the body. All these go further to support the need to eat a variety so we can obtain the maximum potential benefits of flavonoids to our bodies.

In a study conducted in Europe, exploring a variety of flavonoids (including kaempferol, myricetin, and quercetin) and their effect on the risk of Type 2 diabetes, it was found that dietary intake of these flavonoids is consistent in various degrees with a decrease in the risk of type 2 diabetes.[2] This study supports the fact that each of these flavonoids can add up to enhance a health benefit, whether it's in its anti-inflammatory, antioxidation, or simply any benefit that it may have. More so, their varying modes of action help to add varying but equally helpful ways of sometimes solving the same problem. This eventually makes the overall result even better in terms of an enhanced effect.

The little drops matter and make a difference in the long-term overall big picture of your health, so do not take those lightly. There are many studies that show an association between a high intake of foods rich in flavonoids and a consequential decrease in the risk of certain diseases, even certain cancers. A high consumption of flavonoids from various foods, as well as some from black tea, can be associated with a decreased risk of ovarian cancer.[3,4] In these studies, there is a reflection in the way each flavonoid contributes in its own unique way to decrease a particular risk, even when several individual flavonoids eventually do the same. Thus, the more different bases you can cover, the better it is for you in attaining your goal. I continue to emphasize *the importance of quantity, frequency, and variety,* amidst other factors that can potentially contribute to you increasing your intake of fruits and vegetables. Paying attention to some of these factors can significantly help you to increase your intake of flavonoids and help to boost your immune health.

The rich action of many flavonoids against the inflammation process[5] can go a long way to boost your health by fostering some of the processes that equip your body to display better and more effective "fighting" responses. This can be in the form of warding off potential "invaders" (pathogens). It can also be in the form of counteracting the action of certain potential imbalances within the body that could be throwing it off its normal course of good health. Many other attributes of certain flavonoids, as in their "antioxidant" capabilities, and much more, can also feed into enhancing the capabilities of your immune system in defending your body, via some of the concepts described earlier in the book.

Flavonoids are worth our time and attention! Consider challenging yourself in increasing your consumption of certain plant foods, for the benefit of some of these. You'll find it helpful exploring recipes you'd enjoy, using some of these plant foods, so you can go further with eating them. Keep in mind some of the tips I discuss, so you can stay alert to avoiding certain potential pitfalls in certain recipes. Some of these guidelines will come in handy when you need them most, so you're able to make your personal "tweaks" that will aid you to enjoy the full benefits from some of these plant foods. Try to find creative ways that keep you motivated to explore many more plant foods outside of your usual. Do your best to make the most out of these flavonoids in addition to the concepts discussed, and enjoy a long-term success of boosting your immune health, and of course, your overall health.

CHAPTER TWENTY-FOUR

Machines And Oils:
Why The Body?

Just the little amounts you consume will do the trick.

W hen it comes to fats and oils, permit me to use this analogy to drive a few points home. Every good engine needs a lubricant/oil, right? Whether it's your car or your lawn mower, engines need oils to help them maximize their function. The choice of oil is as important as simply putting oil into any engine. It is no wonder when you go for an oil change for your vehicle, you must deal with choosing the "grade" of oil you'd want to use for your vehicle. Higher grade oils tend to attract higher costs. Like the engine of your car, it matters the type of oils you choose to put into your body.

The subject of eating low-fat foods has gotten many caught into believing that they have to avoid eating fats in its totality. This is absolutely not true. This is because it is important to get the benefits from the good fats, without necessarily overloading your body with excessive calories in the process, as good as they are. Generally, fats from plants tend to provide a good source of healthy fats for our bodies. These include fats from avocado, nuts, and seeds, as discussed earlier. In fact, there are certain vitamins, specifically, A, D, E, and K, that are soluble in fats, and whose absorption is enhanced by fats. Just the little amounts you consume will do the trick.

If these fats/oils are that important and all you need are small amounts, then yes, like your vehicle, it matters what kind of fats/oils you put into your body. Remember, that our goal, when it comes to dietary fat consumption, is to consume "good" fats (HDL) in low to moderate quantities, and to drastically decrease the consumption of "bad" fats (LDL). Did you know that in addition to achieving this objective from foods, the oils you use in cooking from your kitchen can help you to do this as well, or in fact, throw you off in the opposite direction?

It is necessary to keep in mind that most cooking oils that stem from most seeds and nuts, generally tend to be a good source of oils for cooking. For example, olive oil, coconut oil, peanut oil, are a few of my popular and most common favorites. Canola oil, originally made from rapeseed plants, continues to be a source of debate with many controversies because of its genetic modification from the original idea of rapeseed that is said to have contained a high amount of erucic acid, known for its potential hazard to health. In an attempt to decrease this erucic acid, the oils continue to be genetically modified and packaged for sale. Be cautious to put health-related information in proper perspective, and do a lot to boost your immune health, so that occasional "junk" choices will not make much of a difference, as your immune system will be in good shape to buffer those infrequent additions.

Many concepts have been shared throughout the book that can help with boosting your immune health. Putting these in practice will help you to be a good user of health-related information. Using these concepts will help you to not live as one always in fear of every negative health news, tossed about by the wind. In fact, knowing the right kind of oils to stock your kitchen with, and how to use them, can go a long way to boost your health.

What should greatly influence your choice of oils at any time in your kitchen is the purpose of your cooking. For example, deep frying versus sautéing. As a general tip in this light, your oven can help you to stay creative in getting many effects of deep-fried foods without actually deep frying them. Find baked and broiled recipes that provide alternatives to deep-fried recipes, keeping in mind the right kinds of oil to use in lightly spraying when desired.

When at all you want to occasionally deep fry, your choice of oils can make a big difference. This is because different oils have different smoking points. Having knowledge about the smoking point of the oils you use in your kitchen is key to using them to the advantage of your health. An oil's smoking point is the temperature at which the oil begins to burn and expel smoke. At this temperature, any potential health benefit contained in this oil to your health has been destroyed. Not only that, the by-product fumes generated from this smoking oil are potentially harmful to the body. Free radicals are also generated from the smoke, which by now, we know to keep them low within our bodies when at all possible. Remember that our goal is to scavenge free radicals from our bodies, so we can boost our immune health. Adding these free radicals to our intake in ways that can easily be prevented is sure not a path we should travel.

For the same reason of the possibility of releasing free radicals in higher quantities at extremely high temperatures, it's needful to consume smoked foods in minimal quantities, so we can decrease the potential of introducing these into the body frequently. Additionally, certain smoked foods are infused with smoke flavor and not the actual smoke, even further complicating the potential of exposing the body to these high amounts of free radicals. Do your best possible to consume smoked foods minimally.

Let me share with you the average smoking points of some of the common oils, refined and unrefined, in our kitchens. Keep in mind that generally, the refined oil equivalents tend to have the higher ends whenever a range in smoking points is indicated, as they have undergone "refinement" to remove some of the content, and which would otherwise cause smoke at a slightly lower temperature. Temperatures are in degree Fahrenheit[1]:

- Canola Oil: 400
- Avocado oil: 520
- Butter: 302
- Coconut oil: 350-400
- Olive oil: 374-470
- Vegetable oil blend: 428
- Peanut oil: 450
- Grapeseed oil: 392

With these in mind, in selecting oils for cooking, it is necessary to consider the temperatures at which you'll be cooking, as well as the types of oils that have more "good fats" versus "bad fats". Oils like corn oil have high proportions of trans fat, despite their high smoke point of a little over 400. For this reason, most people choose to stay away from it. Unfortunately, this, as well as others with similar characteristics tend to be prevalent in the fast food industry. Due to their low cost, in addition to other factors, these are attractive to the fast food industry, although not the same to the body's health.

This is further worsened by the frequent reuse of these oils in deep frying. Every time these oils used for deep frying are used again, they become even more degraded, more gets absorbed into the foods during cooking, potentially contributing to more weight gain, higher cholesterol intake, and higher blood pressure in certain consumers. All these factors contribute immensely to the development of type 2 diabetes and heart disease.[2]

Consuming minimal amounts of fast foods is essential to staying in good health. Of those listed, some of the popular oils that are rich in "good" fats include avocado oil, olive oil, and coconut oil, to mention a few. Extra Virgin Olive oil is wonderful when drizzled in salads and widely used in at home Italian and store-bought Italian salad dressing recipes. Coconut oils tend to increase both HDL ("good" fats) and LDL ("bad" fats), with a resulting "neutralizing effect" unlike most that would only increase "bad" fats. For this reason, it tends to be a great choice, as is olive oil, for quick sautéing, which typically tends to use relatively lower temperatures compared to deep frying. Coconut oil is great for skin and hair health as well, and many women like myself, explore its amazing benefits.

When it comes to deep frying, my ideal recommendation is to keep it very minimal in your diet. In fact, it has been shown from research that people who eat high amounts of fried foods may be at a higher risk of having heart disease and type 2 diabetes.[3] In this study, it was found that people who consumed fried foods once weekly had a higher risk of developing type 2 diabetes and heart disease as compared to people who ate fried foods less than once per week. They found this risk to increase, as the frequency of consuming fried foods weekly increased.

Consistent with our *concept of moderation*, and occasionally eating a little bit of these foods, you'll realize that we may occasionally like to eat little amounts of fried foods. What we do even on those occasions matter and can make a difference also in our overall health. On those rare days when you choose to eat some deep-fried foods, minimizing the frequency of trips to the fast food restaurant may be worth the choice. There are certainly days when you may want to make those trips, and that's okay. The frequency is what you should keep an eye on. The lesser it is, the better, say once bi-weekly, or even lesser. Purposefully planning for those days can help greatly in being successful with your intended choices.

Choosing oils with high smoking points is ideal for deep frying. Peanut oil is a great oil of for deep frying. However, for most people, the cost is prohibitive. Canola oil tends to be one that is common, and reasonably priced. Although the smoking point for canola oil is not as high as that of peanut oil, it is okay to occasionally opt for it as substitute, given all the other factors under consideration. In an occasional deep frying "venture", and with abundant immune health-boosting foods on your table, that infrequent choice in favor of cost would not be a big deal, as in occasional junk food consumption.

Avocado oil is rich in healthy fats, and is another oil of choice when it comes to basic cooking. However, its cost tends to be high as well, and going for olive oil is equally beneficial, when presented with options.

There are many great oils out there, although many less common, but with great health benefits. I hope this discussion gives you a broad idea of what oils to consider with knowledge of their smoking points, and based on the type of cooking you may choose at any given time. Exploring oils, especially with your health at heart, will help you to take advantage of some of the nourishing oils around you, in order to achieve your immune health-boosting objectives. Remember also, that excessive consumption of fats still add extra calories. Keep your overall nutrition in proper perspective, and consume fats in low to moderate quantities, being sure to consume "healthy" fats, and decrease the consumption of "bad" fats. Doing so will help you a long way in staying consistent with strategies that can help in boosting your overall health.

CHAPTER TWENTY-FIVE

Mix Right, Further The Boost

*"Listening" to your body will help you
stay away from what the "masses" do
and do what is best for you.*

W hat came to mind when you first saw this topic? When it comes to foods, many times, making the right picks and pairing with knowledge can further enhance the potential benefits they can contribute to boosting your health. The kind of knowledge that increases your ability and skill to pair right can enhance your food choices and their impact on your health.

Let me use cooking and taste to elaborate on this concept. When you choose to cook in your slow cooker, you realize the first step toward a great outcome is in your ability to choose the right and finest ingredients that go together. You then allow time for these ingredients to intermix, complement, and enhance each other's ability to bring out the desired great taste. When this process is allowed to successfully complete, you can have a better outcome in terms of the taste, than you would have had, should you have eaten any of these cooked foods individually. This applies to stove top cooking as well, but I use the slow cooker concept to bring out an idea of the time given to allow for the ingredients to intermix. When it comes to cooking, you realize that the knowledge you have about the ingredients you choose and how well they intermix with each other can bring about a huge transformation in terms of the resulting taste of your cooked food. That, in turn, can make a huge difference between good and bad cooking. You also realize that acquiring this kind of knowledge is one that spans a lifetime and requires willingness and openness to pursuit.

Now, this is the same when it comes to "pairing and mixing right" to enhance our health in relation to boosting our immune health. Research is ongoing and continues to bring out the knowledge about many foods which when paired appropriately with others, have their health benefits further enhanced. My goal is to introduce this concept using some examples, and to increase your desire to stay open to learning more about these foods. You can use them to your advantage.

Let me start by using some simple but oftentimes overlooked examples. Did you know that many times, lots of the nutrients from some of the foods we eat are not able to make it successfully into our bloodstream because they encounter challenges during the digestive process in terms of absorption? In certain instances, most of the nutrients are not absorbed in terms of quantities, or in amounts we would have loved to have been absorbed. I have mentioned this concept in various discussions in terms of bioavailability (the quantity of nutrients from the foods we eat, or even medications we take, that become usefully available within the bloodstream or body). My goal is to help you to understand how pairing right, or mixing right, based on knowledge can further your effort in eating right.

Did you know that iron absorption is enhanced in an environment rich in Vitamin C? There are certain people who experience low iron levels along with its consequences, not because they do not eat iron-rich foods. There are some who even take iron supplements based on a recommendation from their primary physician. However, they are not able to enjoy its benefits because their bodies are not able to absorb much during digestion.

Many of the vegetables rich in iron tend to be rich also in Vitamin C. For example, for about a 100g of spinach, there is about 2.7 mg of iron, and a corresponding roughly 27 mg of Vitamin C (these estimates are only to give you an idea of what I mean). However, your iron intake from your proteins may not have these corresponding high amounts of Vitamin C, though other conditions make those much easier for the body to absorb in comparison to iron from vegetables, although those tend to have correspondingly high amounts of Vitamin C. Do you see how much of a difference the absorption of iron from your foods could be enhanced simply by filling half your plate with vegetables and fruits as you eat your piece of chicken and baked potatoes?

Don't forget your leafy greens, broccoli, and of course, the various other richly colored fruits and vegetables. These fruits and vegetables tend to be rich in Vitamin C, as well as amazing flavonoids. Making a choice to fill your dinner plate with them can go a long way in enhancing the absorption of a key nutrient, as in iron, from your digestive system. In turn, adequate amounts of iron in your body can help in ensuring you have the energy you need, to keep up with everyday activities. Let me even throw in the fact that you can even consider going for dark meat chicken or turkey to further boost your iron levels and save yourself from any mental "pressures" of a need to eat red meat frequently for iron boosts in your body.

Are you wondering why the extensive elaboration on iron? Iron is a very important element in the body, and roughly 70% of iron in the body can be found in the red blood cells contained in the blood (in a complex called hemoglobin), and in the cells of the muscles called myoglobin. The major function of hemoglobin is to carry oxygen from your lungs when you breathe, to various parts of the body through a system of actions, and to bring carbon dioxide from these bodily parts, back to the lungs. When you breathe out, you get rid of the carbon dioxide. The blood also carries essential nutrients absorbed from the intestines to various parts of the body by other series of actions. Iron plays very crucial functions in the body. When your body does not have enough iron to carry out these needed functions, you begin to feel tired unnecessarily. In certain extreme cases, as this worsens, brain cells could also be deprived of sufficient oxygen and nutrients, and some people get confused. Eventually, various other organs can be impacted.

The body has a system of organs that are very much interconnected and interdependent on each other in terms of ability to function adequately. On the contrary, too much iron intake is dangerous to the body. Your intake from foods is the best and safest way of consuming iron. This method will typically not lead to excessive ingestion. This challenge of excess can typically result when people take iron supplements without a recommendation from their physician.

There are tons of potential causes of fatigue in the body, some of which are not due to low iron intake. For this reason, it is always important to consult your doctor when you have unusual feelings, as in unexplainable fatigue. However, paying attention to your daily nutritional intake by being careful to pair and mix right to enhance iron absorption, can go a long way in making a huge difference in your health, and ensuring you have adequate amounts of iron within, needed for your body's function. There are various other nutrients whose absorption can be further enhanced in an environment with certain other nutrients, making them more available within the body for its use.

There are many other foods that complement each other. Did you know that the absorption of calcium is enhanced by Vitamin D? There are many controversies and opinions when it comes to consuming dairy products. It's always important to consider the *ideas of benefits versus disadvantages, quality, and moderation,* as pertaining to your peculiar circumstances, when confronted with a situation of making certain food choices. This is particularly helpful in the case of certain foods with peculiar controversies as discussed, and will be helpful to you in making a decision that will best suit you under any circumstances.

When it comes to calcium from dairy, I personally hold to a concept of limiting my intake to about a single serving from quality milk products a day, obtaining other servings of Vitamin D and calcium from the sun, my greens, and occasional minimal supplements when needed. This works best for me. I also understand situations where certain individuals cannot consume dairy because of possible allergic reactions or other personal reasons. That's unique to them, as every individual is unique, and "listening" to your body will help you to stay away from what the "masses" do and do what is best for you. The way you choose to consume your calcium is very important because you have an option to maximize your benefits by "pairing right".

Eating high calcium-containing foods alongside rich Vitamin D-containing foods or sources can help to boost absorption of the calcium. This can then heighten the benefits you could potentially obtain from them, such as strong teeth and bones, and much more, even in terms of your body's functional performance. I mentioned milk because many calcium-rich products also contain Vitamin D. Vitamin D has enormous benefits, and adequate intake is essential. Many studies have shown that low Vitamin D intake increases the risk of many diseases such as certain cancers, heart disease, certain bone diseases both in children and adults, and much more.[1]

Bear in mind the Recommended Daily Intake when using supplements (Tip: read labels on bottles), while also knowing that some portions may not be totally absorbed into your bloodstream, from your digestive system. Eating a balanced diet rich in vegetables and fruits can help you to further achieve your recommended daily intake of vitamins and minerals. Your occasional supplements only help to fill potential gaps. Remember, these nutrients are best absorbed in foods, a reason why taking your supplements with food will help enhance absorption.

A simple exposure to the sun for 10 minutes a day can go a long way to make a difference in getting your daily recommended intake of Vitamin D. There are also potential exposures to UV radiations from the sun, for which precautions must be taken to decrease potential dangers. These precautions can include using an effective sunscreen, choosing appropriate protective clothing and gear, as well as choosing to stay out in the sun during a decent time of the day when UV radiation emission is low. When these precautions are in place, you can obtain immense benefits from the sun.

Your doctor usually monitors your Vitamin D levels together with certain other tests when you go for your annual checkups, to make sure you are keeping up with your body's needs of those. I threw this example into this discussion to further support the *concept of moderation*, knowing *benefits versus disadvantages*, and *balance*, when making food-related health choices. It is dangerous to make decisions based on partial information, especially based on your knowledge of potential negatives only, without understanding potential benefits as well as any precautionary

measures you could take to prevent experiencing potential negatives while obtaining optimal benefits from the positives. I
hope this understanding helps you the next time you are faced
with a decision like whether or not to get sun exposure, or even
eat a particular vegetable or food.

This concept gets even better and more interesting. I used
the examples from the Vitamin D and iron to foster an initial
understanding because they are very common and easy to relate
to. My main objective is to help you to solidify an understanding of the importance of staying knowledgeable when it comes
to "pairing and mixing right" to further boost your effort to stay
in good health. From the discussion of Turmeric (Chapter 14),
you'll notice that like many other foods, I mention the challenge
with getting lots of the nutrients from it available in the bloodstream (bioavailability) due to absorption challenges. With that
said, a study has shown that a significant nutrient in black pepper spice known as Bioperine, in addition to its own benefits,
can also help to enhance absorption of certain nutrients and
vitamins from the gut, including turmeric.[2]

Currently, lots of research studies have not been devoted
solely to the study of Bioperine, but the few out there give us a
good indication of its enhanced absorption capability. I believe
we will begin to see more research studies devoted to Bioperine
in the future. Hopefully, this helps you to consider sprinkling
some more black pepper on your food, the next time you are at
a restaurant or eating at the dinner table, most especially if you
are tempted to sprinkle some extra salt. Skipping that extra salt
and adding extra black pepper instead, can go a long way to help
boost your immune health.

When it comes to not eating certain foods because of the
possible dangers they pose, some potential dangers could be decreased on those occasional days when we crave for them, by

simply pairing right based on knowledge. With the *concept of 85% or more healthy and 15% or less occasional "junk,"* you'll see that even on that occasional 15% "junk deal", the *concept of moderation* and *pairing right* can come in handy.

A few examples will help to further throw light on this concept. For example, rosmarinic acid in certain plants from the mint family such as rosemary and oregano, will help to decrease the formation of certain potential carcinogens (substances/compounds with a potential of causing cancer in living tissue) such as heterocyclic amines, which are otherwise produced when red meat is exposed to high temperatures during cooking.[3] This reduction could be as high as 71%.[4] It would be helpful keeping in mind that your occasional hamburger or beef treat could be a reality without the feeling of guilt, simply by adding a generous amount of rosemary and oregano to your lean hamburger patty mixes before you fire them up on your grill. Plus, you get an additional bonus from the added rich taste.

Let me go yet another step. You know how sometimes you stay away from certain occasional treats, whether it's from your favorite Chinese restaurant or some other restaurant because you are unsure of whether or not MSG (monosodium glutamate)-containing seasonings have been used excessively in cooking their foods. You know when it comes to most restaurants, they focus on you getting great tastes from their foods so they can keep you coming back as a life-long customer. Many times, the goal of trying to keep happy customers gets in the way of making healthy ingredient choices during cooking, amidst other factors. For you, your concern may be trying to ensure you're keeping your health in great shape while also enjoying certain foods, so you can stay productive and enjoy your life for a longer period. You may be aware of certain potential hazards of MSG-containing seasonings to the body's health. Unfortunately, MSG can be found in many commercially prepared foods, both cooked and uncooked. Many times, restaurant-prepared foods are no exception, and it becomes a concern for many who want to stay away from MSG.

So, imagine you are eating this hot delicious meal you just ordered at the restaurant, but have all these guilt trails in your mind that could be keeping you from enjoying your meal because you have potential concerns about MSG. What do you do? Let me tell you that this is another instance where pairing and mixing right based on knowledge can keep the guilt away and get you on your way to enjoying that occasional treat.

We do know that Vitamin C can reduce or even prevent the potentially negative effects of MSG as in headaches.[5] Under such circumstance, I believe that having ensured that at least 85% of your week's intake has been geared toward eating foods that have empowered your immune system to "fight" potential "hazards" (as in MSG in this instance) would be a good place to have started from. Simply throwing in extra Vitamin C-rich sides and additions to your meal then, as in some freshly squeezed lemons in your water, eating your fruits and vegetables, etc. will help you to enjoy your meal guilt-free. What you eat the 85% of the time of your week or month can positively or negatively impact the health of your immune system, based on your choices.

Furthermore, pairing and mixing right, as well as being moderate, can help you to enjoy eating guilt-free even on those occasional "junk days". A proper application of this concept can help you to enjoy your life while making sure those "feel- good" hormones (see Chapter 7) are secreted in high amounts to even further your immune health boost strides.

In conclusion, let me say that many times, the health benefit of one plant food can be further enhanced by another, a major reason why pairing and mixing right can make a huge difference in your health. Even with the use of essential oils, those familiar with them will realize that in certain instances, you'll find mixes that further enhance the property being explored.

For example, in a study exploring the antibacterial property of plants in treating *E. Coli* (*Escherichia coli*) in the case of Irritable Bowel Syndrome, it was found that mixes were most potent, with a mixture of coriander, lemon balm, and mint.[6] As individuals, each of these different plants has some antibacterial properties, but together, they can do so much more. There are many bioactive compounds that span across similar plants, as well as many multiples that tend to occur in singular plants. It is no wonder many can complement and enhance each other's effect, as even in many of the spices we use in our cooking.

I could go extensively into illustrating with many more examples, but my goal is to help you to understand this concept and stir within you a lifelong desire and openness to acquiring even more knowledge on specifics, when it comes to making your food choices. Doing this will go a long way in helping you to provide that additional boost your health will benefit from, while also enjoying your precious life.

CHAPTER TWENTY-SIX

The "Petite" Questions

*In boosting your health, it's important to
stay engaged and informed, and be willing
to find out what works best for you.*

I kept in mind those little questions I thought might have baffled your mind as you read the book. I try to address these in this concluding chapter, hoping they will help you to further believe you can do what it takes in applying some of the discussed concepts to the long-term success of enhancing your health. My whole focus has been on empowering you with foundational concepts that will well-position you to boost your immune health.

I have also explored the world of foods, especially plant foods, via the area of spices and other pertinent foods, in ways that should challenge you to take advantage of them in boosting your health, as eating is one of the basic everyday things we do to help with our sustenance. Boosting your immune health with simple, but many times overlooked plant foods from the center of your home while practicing some of these valuable concepts discussed, will help you to consistently stir your everyday eating habits in a positive direction. My emphasis in this addition has been on the benefits of certain spices and common foods most of us have in our kitchen but many times tend to underutilize. I hope you've been motivated to look at your kitchen in a whole different way, seeing its potential ability to help boost your immune health or the other way around, based on your choices. Your long-term success in achieving your health goals is important to me. I believe the practice of some of these discussed concepts will help you in achieving long-term success in this aspect of life.

Based on my own experiences and acquired knowledge, I do my best to answer some of your potential questions, and I hope these answers will help you to cement together the usefulness of some of the concepts you've read about throughout the book.

What Has Research To Do With My Health?

Let me talk about this incident which I hope you may be familiar with, as I use certain aspects to further throw light on the role of research in advancing health and healthcare. Do you remember not too long ago, in late 2014, early 2015 when the scare of an Ebola outbreak in certain African countries as in the cases of Liberia and Sierra Leone which were heavily affected, swept across many countries of the world? The fear was predominantly related to the common possible modes of transmission of this virus as via common bodily fluids, said to have included saliva, and even tears. The mode of transmission of this virus, and how quickly an infection from it could result in death, led to many strict ways of isolating infected people and containing the disease in affected areas. Promptly isolating people infected by the virus, among many other derived solutions, led to success in dealing with the outbreak in the long run. During this time, there were many missionaries out in the field, helping to contain and eradicate the outbreak.

I remember so well one that touched my heart and one which I personally prayed for and whose story I closely followed, with a joy of being able to witness the true faithfulness of God in his journey through recovery and cure from the deadly disease. Dr. Ken Brantly of the Samaritan's Purse, an international missionary organization, was on the ground then, actively working in the wake of the outbreak.[1] Dr. Brantly contracted the disease while he worked to save lives. I remember hearing this on the news and immediately began to pray that God would let His glory be revealed through the life of this precious and selfless medical doctor. I prayed and asked God to save his life, and I knew there were many people all over the world whose hearts God would also touch to actively and continually pray in this same manner. God truly healed him, and indeed, it was a miracle, as I followed his story to the very point of great success.

In this remarkable story of Dr. Brantly's healing, I remember an experimental drug called ZMapp, which was a major drug that was administered to him as mentioned in the news, and which stimulated a quick turn onto the paths of healing for this amazing doctor. Until it was tested on Dr. Brantly and another missionary, this drug had only been tested on monkeys.[2, 3] I mention this to elaborate on the importance of laboratory animals and the clues they provide to us in health research. In this story, I believe that God used findings from earlier research studies using ZMapp to help provide clues that would save the life of Dr. Brantly.

There are many ways in which research can impact your health positively. I focus on a narrow aspect of this, specifically as pertaining to boosting your immune health, and consistent with the scope of discussions focused on throughout the book. I mention some research findings with a goal of helping to paint valuable and lasting mental pictures that would consistently influence positive choices. This is because research studies, and within this scope with this aspect of health, can many times solve many "mysteries" that have presented themselves as barriers to the well-being of humans. Whether it's in exploring the cure for a disease, or simply finding out what little tweaks can be made to positively impact certain potential health challenges, research can provide valuable clues that many times over several years are able to provide pointers to the discovery of certain solutions.

Depending on what type of research is being conducted, there can be various stages and phases in a research "cycle". For example, when it comes to exploring let's say a cure for a disease, in the most initial phase, the use of experimental animals is explored. Various types of these experimental animals can be used, with some popular ones being guinea pigs and laboratory rats. Without going into extensive detail, these animals are used initially for various ethical and safety reasons that would prohibit the use of humans.

Of course, think about the fact that certain diseased cells obtained for experimental use in these animals are many times replicated intentionally, and various experimental factors are manipulated. Many ambiguities, as in this, and the uncertainty of outcomes, would prohibit initial testing in humans. However, over time, as possible clues are found and safety measures are considered, possible experimental treatment pathways are developed for testing in humans. These experimental studies are carried out in human subjects who already have the conditions being considered, ensuring that certain defined measures, safety measures, and protocols are closely adhered to.

Disease conditions are not replicated experimentally in humans, but should already exist for any study. Many other considerations are made, prior to carrying out experimental studies involving human subjects. Finding the right and safe amounts of whatever potential treatment substance is being tested in humans, can also pose a challenge, and that is typically found over several repetitions of experiments using various amounts, initially in experimental animals, to find those safe dosages. Due to these and many other challenges including cost amidst others, many times, it generally takes a considerably long time before any helpful studies are conducted in human subjects.

It is important to know there can be safe ways of using these experimental research findings relating to food, no matter what stage or phase of the research these findings come from in terms of "breaking through". When it comes to the subject of studying the benefits of food components, most of these foods we already eat, we know are typically safe for consumption. This assumes you have no allergies to them, have considered quality standards in purchasing them, are eating them in safe food quantities, and of course, have considered any other safety parameters that are pertinent to your specific situation.

While using experimental research animals, various additional clues can be obtained with regards to certain benefits of certain foods to health. Information from some of these research findings can give us clues to know which foods we should purposefully consider consuming more of. You can take advantage of some of these clues, and use them safely to your advantage, especially with regards to foods that are so easily obtainable, and many of which you are already eating and could simply increase frequency of consumption, to obtain additional benefits. This is a major way information from research findings can become very useful in practice, to us. It is worth having knowledge of health research findings. This kind of knowledge can be invaluable to your health. It will help you to make choices that can enhance your health.

There are many people who try to enrich what they eat with certain food supplements. I also do this occasionally, depending on my need. This is because sometimes it is difficult, most especially on certain days, for me to meet the daily required amounts of certain key nutrients. When I use supplements, I base my use on knowledge obtained from extensive research and experience.

Let me throw in a general word of caution when it comes to using food supplements. First, remember to discuss use with your physician, as certain supplements may interact with, decrease the efficacy of, increase the efficacy of, etc., of certain prescribed medications. Dosage, quality, and many other factors that pertain to your specific situations are only a few more factors to consider when acquiring knowledge, and when speaking to your physician.

Consider discussing the length of time of use of supplements when acquiring knowledge and conversing with your physician. This is because certain supplements present dangers when used beyond certain periods and may not be safe for long-term use. It is important to always put your safety at the heart of any decisions you make. Starting slowly and staying informed is helpful with any new thing. Your health is no exception to this rule. Stay informed, acquire lots of knowledge, consult with your healthcare professionals, and stay on top of decisions that impact your health. Research findings can greatly help to increase your knowledge and can help you make choices that can potentially boost your health.

Why Is It Working For Mr. A But Not For Me?

This is a very common question many people ask themselves with regards to foods and other regimens, and I thought to discuss that, to help you stay focused and on track, should you be asking this same question. When it comes to the body, everyone's body is made up of unique genetic components. Genetics play an important function in what makes each one of us unique, and can sometimes influence disease processes in certain individuals, although environmental factors can contribute to this as well. Even our fingerprints are not the same. Not only are our fingerprints not the same, but they are unique, and never like anyone else's. God is indeed wonderful! This genetic makeup, in turn, impacts our physiological makeup. These specific genetic compositions, as well as many other factors, like environmental factors, can sometimes inter-relate to produce an effect. Some of these effects can include allergic reactions to certain foods or substances in certain individuals, which other people may not necessarily experience under similar conditions. In some people, some of these allergic reactions may be occasional, seasonal, or even extend through their lifespan.

Because of our different and unique make ups, some things that work for others may not necessarily work for us. Even medications! Foods tend to follow this general pattern as well. Imagine some of the noticeable differences we may have, as in even our weight differences. I use weight here because sometimes, even certain medications are adjusted to accommodate differences in weight. I mention this to paint the picture that it is very possible for some things including certain foods, to work for some people but not necessarily us, for various reasons. However, we can strive to find what works for us only if we keep trying. There are many options, and the right knowledge can provide us with valuable pointers.

Think about the many different possible ways of meeting let's say, a nutritional requirement. For example, someone may have allergies to dairy products but can meet all their nutritional calcium requirements through the consumption of green leafy vegetables, almonds, and various other foods rich in calcium, without a need to consume dairy products.

I pause to simply say God is all-wise, and he has made room for each one of us to stay in health, no matter our preferences or health challenges, as in the allergies example I mentioned.

On the flip side also, although research has, and continues to provide clues to certain natural remedies, unique individual physiological differences can present a barrier that would typically prevent anyone in many instances, from rushing to make statements applicable to a general population, simply based on research findings using a sample of the general population. Furthermore, there are typically potential limitations that can be present in any research study. Keep in mind, that this should not stop us from obtaining clues that could potentially help us in our individual situations. These unique differences amidst other factors prohibit quick generalizations despite positive clues.

For example, the American Diabetes Association (ADA) may well recognize that cinnamon has been beneficial to certain diabetics in helping to regulate their blood sugar[4]. However, for the fact that results from certain other studies have not replicated the same results amidst other factors, the ADA refrains from recommending cinnamon as a blood glucose regulator to its general population of diabetics with varying physiologies and many other differences. It would be difficult to tell who would benefit from, and who may not, as in the variations with certain study findings. This is the right thing to do, given the wide range of diabetic population ADA serves, so someone doesn't misinterpret such information and abolish any recommended diet, medication, or lifestyle changes for their specific situation, in pursuit of cinnamon as a supposed cure for their diabetic condition.

Does this stance nullify the possibility that for certain people, occasional consumption of cinnamon may regulate their blood sugar levels? Of course not! Again, different things may work well or better for different people, and other foods may work better for some people than cinnamon (as you can see from some of our discussions, there is a wide variety of foods that may help with the body's ability to regulate its blood sugar). What am I saying? I'm simply saying, that it is very possible for a diabetic to work closely with their healthcare provider in monitoring the progression of their health, with any dietary and lifestyle changes they choose to make. For example, with the cinnamon, a choice to consume in food-safe quantities, stay within prescribed regimens, and with all other safety boundaries as defined by their physician in place, a person could work closely with their physician to monitor the impact of their choice of cinnamon consumption on their blood sugar regulation. Their physician can work with them to tailor their medications to fit outcomes.

This requires time, willingness to try various foods and other lifestyle changes, while working closely with your health care provider and other professionals, to find what changes work best for you in your specific situation. Taking an approach of eating in food-safe quantities of any foods that are tried is needful. Your safety is always important and should be at the heart of all your actions.

For these reasons and many others, I encourage you to find what works best for you, and not be discouraged by the fact that what has worked for someone else has not worked for you. I can tell you that even with medications, I have seen certain ones work for certain people and not others. Your willingness to keep trying is the simplest key that could potentially unlock what works best for you.

Never give up, especially when it comes to making right food picks and your health. You can overcome your challenges. I hope reading this book has encouraged you to know that there is plenty of room for you to experience good health by making informed choices that will boost your immune health.

When it comes to boosting your immune health, it's important to consider staying engaged and informed. Be willing to explore what works best for you. Gleaning from the experiences of other people will also help you locate clues as you work on finding what works best for you. Practice the concepts discussed throughout this book and remember to eat a wide variety of health-boosting foods. And finally, consider including some of the amazing immune health-boosting foods discussed in this book to help accelerate your path to better health.

Welcome to a new *Healthy Me*!

GLOSSARY

Anticarcinogens: substances that have an ability to negate the effects of carcinogens (substances that are capable of causing cancer in living tissue). Hence, in a broad sense, carcinogens are generally also referred to as substances with potential cancer preventive capabilities.

Antiemetic: a substance with an ability to prevent vomiting.

Antioxidants: Substances that prevent oxidation. Oxidation is the loss of electron from an unstable molecule, atom, ion, etc., This can lead to highly reactive chemical reactions, which, in turn can cause damage in the process within the body. Antioxidants can prevent these oxidative reactions from taking place by creating more stable molecules. Also, antioxidants can work to "scavenge" potentially toxic free radicals, thus disarming them of their harmful effects and detoxifying the body.

Flavonoids: compounds in plants that are of benefit to health.

Free radicals: highly charged molecules, that can easily react with other molecules such as those normal molecules within the body, and cause damage to them.

Gram-negative and Gram-positive bacteria: These are two major groupings generally used for differentiating bacteria based on the variations shown in their cell walls, using a type of test known as the Gram stain test. In this test, bacteria are stained using a special "dye". In response to this test, the bacteria would show to be either gram-positive or gram-negative.

The Gram-positive bacteria have relatively thicker cell walls and retain the color of the "dye", showing a purple coloration when seen under a microscope; on the contrary, gram-negative bacteria have thin walls and do not retain the dye's color, but reflect a pinkish coloration when observed under a microscope.

HDL: High-density lipoproteins, commonly known as HDLs or "good cholesterol" or "good fats".

Homeostasis: an ability of the body to seek and maintain a stable internal condition when dealing with changes in its external environment.

LDL: Low-density lipoproteins, commonly known as LDLs, "bad cholesterol" or "bad fats".

Oxidative stress: can occur in the body when an imbalance is created because the body's rate of production of free radicals is much higher than its ability to counteract, get rid of, or detoxify the harmful effects created by the presence of these free radicals.

Pathogen: A microorganism such as a virus or bacteria that has an ability to cause disease.

Peristalsis/Peristaltic movements: an involuntary contraction and relaxation of the muscles of the intestines, that provide a wave-like motion which moves food along the tract during digestion.

Polyphenols: a group of micronutrients in certain foods, that afford them high antioxidant properties.

LIST OF KEY WELLNESS CONCEPTS

Here are a few of the key derived Wellness Concepts I discussed along with their extensive variations in application, together with "Immune-Strengthening" tactics:

Concept of:

i. *Balance*

ii. *Moderation*

iii. *Staying physically active*

iv. *Being "boss of your body"*

v. *Gratification-at-will*

vi. *The minimum of 85:15 "healthy versus unhealthy" foods ratio*

vii. *Pairing right*

viii. *Benefits versus disadvantages*

AUTHOR'S NOTES

Introducing My Personal Friend

Let me introduce to you my amazing, personal friend who makes all the difference in my life. His name is Jesus! If you do not know Him personally yet and have not accepted him as your Lord and Savior, no worries at all. I can help. I have come to realize that sometimes life can take a toll on you, and the help of a personal friend in the journey is priceless. I treasure the help of this friend and speak to Him before I start my day, every day. He is with me always during the day to help me through any challenges I face. If you do not already know Him, I encourage you to take a moment to take these very simple steps:

History lets us know from the bible that we are all sinners, and none of us is righteous because of the sins of Adam and Eve. We all are born sinners. Jesus Christ died for our sins, and anyone who believes that he or she is a sinner and Christ died for his or her sins, and confesses Jesus Christ as his or her personal savior would be saved (Romans 10:8,9; John 3:16, The NKJV Bible). You see, it sounds simple, but it made a huge difference in my life, and it can happen for you too!

If you believe also in your heart, take a moment, pause, and confess this with your lips: Lord Jesus, I believe today that I am a sinner and that Christ Jesus came to die for my sins. I invite you today into my heart and life to be my personal savior and friend. Thank you, in Jesus' name I pray. Amen!

Yes, it's that easy. You have a new personal friend in your life, I rejoice with you, and I know without a shadow of a doubt that He will help you in your health like He's helping me with mine. Find a Bible-believing church family near you, and let the pastor know about the confession you just made, and he will help you to connect deeper with this new friend. Feel free to contact me if you need assistance finding a Bible-believing church near you, and I'll be glad to help.

Now, this is the friend I talk to every morning before I start my day. I started by setting aside 10 minutes each day, and I realize now that the time frame has grown with time, as I look forward to those moments. The chosen time set aside may be different for different people. You could start with 5 minutes if that's all you've got and watch Him do amazing things in your life.

One important thing is being sincere when you talk to Him. Know that even your secrets are safe with Him, that's how great of a friend He is. After I have talked to him, I keep His word in my heart, and throughout the day, I simply believe He's with me, and I talk to Him in my heart, or verbally when alone. I do this, whether I need help solving a problem with work, or making decisions when confronted with choices. If you've taken the simple step to accept Him, or you already know Him, believe He is with you, talk to Him about everything during the day, from the dog to your difficult boss. He understands and will help you in various ways. Sometimes He'll help you through people and circumstances, other times, He will put great thoughts and ideas in your mind as you think about His word. I also talk to Him when I feel disappointed. This is very helpful to me, knowing that there is someone I can always talk to, and it helps in keeping me from feeling overwhelmed and nurturing chronic stress.

Finally, let me ask this: Are you or a loved one struggling with a health condition? This friend you've just accepted into your life can help you, just like He helped me. He continues to help me and many others. He has the power and ability to heal even in the worst of situations. If you are in desperate need of God's healing power, I pray for you, that God will come through in meeting this need of healing. I also pray for you, that He will show you the steps you need to take to experience His healing, in the mighty name of Jesus!

Chapter Notes

Chapter 2 - Arm Your Body Right

1. Perkins, A. (1994). Saving money by reducing stress. *Harvard Business Review*, 72(6), 12.

2. Psalm 37:8 NKJV.

3. The Centers for Disease Control and Prevention (2017). Health Effects of Chemical Exposure. Retrieved from https://www.atsdr.cdc.gov/emes/public/docs/health%20effects%20of%20chemical%20exposure%20fs.pd. (accessed March 8th, 2017).

Chapter 3 - A Scavenger Hunt Within: Aim For This!

1. Rajendran, P., Nandakumar, N., Rengarajan, T., Palaniswami, R., Gnanadhas, E.N., Lakshminarasaiah, U., Gopas, J., Nishigaki, I. (2014). Antioxidants and human diseases. *Clinica Chimica Acta*, 436, 332-347. Doi: 10.1016/j.cca.2014.06.004.

2. Pham-Huy, L. A., He, H., & Pham-Huy, C. (2008). Free Radicals, Antioxidants in Disease and Health. *International Journal of Biomedical Science*, 4(2), 89–96.

3. Gutman, J. (2002). *GSH Your Body's Most Powerful Protector Glutathione* (3rd ed.). Communications Kudo. ca Inc., Montreal.

4. National Institutes of Health, office of Dietary Supplements (2018). Vitamin C, Fact Sheet for Health Professionals. Retrieved from https://ods.od.nih.gov/factsheets/VitaminC-HealthProfessional/.

5. National Cancer Institute (2018). High-Dose Vitamin C (PDQ)- Patient Version. Retrieved from https://www.cancer.gov/about-cancer/treatment/cam/patient/vitamin-c-pdq#link/_18.

6. Ibid, 5.

7. Ibid, 5.

Chapter 4 - Put Out The Little Fires

1. Pratheeshkumar, P., Son, Y.-O., Budhraja, A., Wang, X., Ding, S., Wang, L., ... Shi, X. (2012). Luteolin Inhibits Human Prostate Tumor Growth by Suppressing Vascular Endothelial Growth Factor Receptor 2-Mediated Angiogenesis. *PLoS ONE*, 7(12), e52279, Doi: 10.1371/journal.pone.0052279.

2. American Heart Association (2016). Inflammation and Heart Disease. Retrieved from http://www.heart.org/HEARTORG/Conditions/Inflammation-and-Heart-Disease_UCM_432150_Article.jsp#.WAUZZ-grKhc on 10/17/2016 (accessed on October 17th, 2016).

3. Wellen, K. E., & Hotamisligil, G. S. (2005). Inflammation, stress, and diabetes. *Journal of Clinical Investigation*, 115(5), 1111–1119. Doi: 10.1172/JCI200525102.

4. Ozcan U, et al. (2004). Endoplasmic reticulum stress links obesity, insulin action, and type 2 diabetes.

American Association For The Advancement of Science, 306 (5695), 457-461.

5. Chen, A. Y., & Chen, Y. C. (2013). A review of the dietary flavonoid, kaempferol on human health and cancer chemoprevention. *Food Chemistry*, 138(4), 2099–2107. Doi: 10.1016/j.foodchem.2012.11.139.

Chapter 5 - What Fuels the Fires?

1. Wikipedia Contributors (2017). Fire Extinguisher, In *Wikipedia, The Free Encyclopedia*. Retrieved from https://en.wikipedia.org/wiki/Fire_extinguisher (accessed May 11th, 2017).

2. Boone, J.L. & Anthony, J.P. (2003). Evaluating the impact of stress on systemic disease: the MOST protocol in primary care. *The Journal of The American Osteopathic Association*, 103(5), 239-246.

3. 3. Psych Central (2018). How Does Stress Affect Us? American Psychological Asssociation. Retrieved from http://psychcentral.com/lib/how-does-stress-affect-us/# (accessed on November 7th, 2018).

4. Ibid, 3.

5. Carnegie Mellon University (2012, April 2). How stress influences disease: Study reveals inflammation as the culprit. Retrieved from ScienceDaily website, www.sciencedaily.com/releases/2012/04/120402162546.htm (accessed on February 2nd, 2018).

6. 6. Sheldon C., Denise J.-D., William J. D., Gregory E. M., Ellen F., Bruce S. R., and Ronald B. T. (2012). Chronic stress, glucocorticoid receptor resistance, inflammation, and disease risk. *Proceedings of the National*

Academy of Sciences of the United States of America, April 2, 2012. Doi: 10.1073/pnas.1118355109.

7. Ibid, 5.

8. Ibid, 6.

9. Ibid, 5.

10. Ibid, 6.

Chapter 6 - Killing A Major Enemy: My Personal Experience

1. Philippians 4:13 NKJV.

2. Introducing My Personal Friend.

3. Proverbs 3: 5,6 NKJV.

4. World Health Organization (2016). The WHO definition of Health. Retrieved from http://www.who.int/about/definition/en/print.html (accessed on November, 10th, 2016).

5. Walton RG, Hudak R, Green-Waite RJ. (1993). Adverse reactions to aspartame: double-blind challenge in patients from a vulnerable population. *Journal of the Society of Biological Psychiatry,* 34 (1-2): 13-7.

6. Briffa, J. (2005). Aspartame and its effects on health: Independently funded studies have found potential for adverse effects. *British Medical Journal,* 330 (7486), 309–310.

7. Sánchez-Villegas, A., Verberne, L., De Irala, J., Ruíz-Canela, M., Toledo, E., Serra-Majem, L., & Martínez-González, M. A. (2011). Dietary Fat Intake and the Risk of Depression, The SUN Project, *PLoS ONE,* 6(1), e16268. Doi: 10.1371/journal.pone.0016268.

8. Crawford, G. B., Khedkar, A., Flaws, J. A., Sorkin, J. D., & Gallicchio, L. (2011). Depressive symptoms and self-reported fast-food intake in midlife women. *Preventive Medicine*, 52(3-4), 254–257. Doi: 10.1016/j.ypmed.2011.01.006.

9. Richards, G., & Smith, A. (2015). Caffeine consumption and self-assessed stress, anxiety, and depression in secondary school children. *Journal of Psychopharmacology* (Oxford, England), 29(12), 1236–1247. Doi: 10.1177/0269881115612404.

10. Gilliland K, Andress D. (1981) Ad lib caffeine consumption, symptoms of caffeinism, and academic performance. *The American Journal of Psychiatry*, 138(4), 512–514.

11. Borchard, T. (2015). 7 Foods That May Contribute to Your Depression. Retrieved from Psych Central webite, http://psychcentral.com/blog/archives/2013/07/11/7-foods-that-may-contribute-to-your-depression/ (accessed November 11th, 2016)

12. Fraze,r A., Hensler, J.G. Serotonin Involvement in Physiological Function and Behavior. In: Siegel GJ, Agranoff BW, Albers RW, et al., editors. *Basic Neurochemistry: Molecular, Cellular and Medical Aspects* (6th ed.). Philadelphia: Lippincott-Raven; 1999, https://www.ncbi.nlm.nih.gov/books/NBK27940/ 74 (accessed on May 11th, 2017).

13. www.drugs.com (accessed on March 2nd, 2017)

14. Lomagno, K. A., Hu, F., Riddell, L. J., Booth, A. O., Szymlek-Gay, E. A., Nowson, C. A., & Byrne, L. K. (2014). Increasing Iron and Zinc in Pre-Menopausal Women and Its Effects on Mood and Cognition: A

Systematic Review. *Nutrients*, 6(11), 5117–5141. Doi: 10.3390/nu6115117.

15. Crozier, S. J., Preston, A. G., Hurst, J. W., Payne, M. J., Mann, J., Hainly, L., & Miller, D. L. (2011). Cacao seeds are a "Super Fruit": A comparative analysis of various fruit powders and products. *Chemistry Central Journal*, 5, 5. Doi: 10.1186/1752-153X-5-5.

Chapter 7 - Let The Butterflies Loose

1. Ibid, Chapter 5, #1.

Chapter 8 - Your Swimming Pool: Make It A Fabulous One!

1. The United States Department of Agriculture (2018). Website, https://www.choosemyplate.gov/.

Chapter 9 - Think Physical Activity

1. Centers for Disease Control and Prevention (2018). Physical Activity. Retrieved from https://www.cdc.gov/physicalactivity/basics/adults/.

2. Saito, K., Tanaka, Y., Ota, T., Eto, S., & Yamashita, U. (1991). Suppressive effect of hyperbaric oxygenation on immune responses of normal and autoimmune mice. *Clinical and Experimental Immunology*, 86(2), 322–327.

3. Harch Hyperbaric Oxygen Therapy (2018). Retrieved from www.hbot.com (accessed on May 11th, 2018).

4. Federation of American Societies for Experimental Biology (2013, December 2). Oxygen levels affect

effectiveness of anti-inflammatory therapies. Retrieved from the ScienceDaily website, www.sciencedaily.com/releases/2013/12/131202121536.htm (accessed on March 11th, 2018).

5. DeBoer, L. B., Powers, M. B., Utschig, A. C., Otto, M. W., & Smits, J. A. (2012). Exploring exercise as an avenue for the treatment of anxiety disorders. *Expert Review of Neurotherapeutics*, 12(8), 1011–1022. Doi: 10.1586/ern.12.73.

Chapter 10 - Rest To Gain

1. Meriam-webster.com (2018). Definition of rest. Retrieved from http://www.merriam-webster.com/dictionary/rest.

2. National Sleep Foundation (2018). What Happens When You Sleep? Retrieved from https://sleepfoundation.org/how-sleep-works/what-happens-when-you-sleep.

3. National Heart, Heart, Lung, and Blood Institute (2018). How Much Sleep Is Enough? Retrieved from https://www.nhlbi.nih.gov/health/health-topics/topics/sdd/howmuch.

4. Ibid, 2.

5. Besedovsky, L., Lange, T., & Born, J. (2012). Sleep and immune function. *Pflugers Archiv* (European Journal of Physiology), 463(1), 121–137. Doi: 10.1007/s00424-011-1044-0.

6. American Heart Association (2018). Know your fats. Retrieved from http://www.heart.

org/HEARTORG/Conditions/Cholesterol/
PreventionTreatmentofHighCholesterol/Know-Your-
Fats_UCM_305628_Article.jsp#.

7. American Heart Association (2018). Website, http://
www.heart.org/HEARTORG/.

Chapter 11 - The "Boss Of Your Body"

1. Philippians 4:13 NKJV.

2. 1 Corinthians 6:19-20 NKJV.

Chapter 12 - Spice Up Your Health

1. Xiong, J. S., Branigan, D., & Li, M. (2009).
Deciphering the MSG controversy. *International
Journal of Clinical and Experimental Medicine*, 2(4),
329–336.

2. Centers for Disease Control and Prevention (CDC),
Fourth National Report on Human Exposure to
Environmental Chemicals (2009), https://www.cdc.
gov/exposurereport/pdf/fourthreport.pdf (accessed on
May 11th, 2017).

Chapter 13 – Ginger

1. Jolad S.D., Lantz R.C., Solyom A.M., Chen G.J.,
Bates R.B., Timmermann, B.N. (2004). Fresh or-
ganically grown ginger (*Zingiber officinale*): composition and effects on LPS-induced PGE2 production.
Phytochemistry, 65(13), 1937-54.

2. Mashhadi, N. S., Ghiasvand, R., Askari, G., Hariri, M., Darvishi, L., & Mofid, M. R. (2013). Anti-Oxidative and Anti-Inflammatory Effects of Ginger in Health and Physical Activity: Review of Current Evidence. *International Journal of Preventive Medicine*, 4(Suppl 1), S36–S42.

3. Park, Y. J., Wen, J., Bang, S., Park, S. W., & Song, S. Y. (2006). [6]-Gingerol Induces Cell Cycle Arrest and Cell Death of Mutant p53-expressing Pancreatic Cancer Cells. *Yonsei Medical Journal*, 47(5), 688–697. Doi: 10.3349/ymj.2006.47.5.688.

4. Prasad, S., & Tyagi, A. K. (2015). Ginger and Its Constituents: Role in Prevention and Treatment of Gastrointestinal Cancer. *Gastroenterology Research and Practice*, 2015, 142979. Doi: 10.1155/2015/142979.

5. Dugasani S., Pichika M.R., Nadarajah V.D., Balijepalli M.K., Tandra S., Korlakunta J.N. (2010). Comparative antioxidant and anti-inflammatory effects of [6]-gingerol, [8]-gingerol, [10]-gingerol and [6]-shogaol. *Journal of Ethnopharmacology*, 127(2), 515–20.

6. Wargovich, M. J., Morris, J., Brown, V., Ellis, J., Logothetis, B., & Weber, R. (2010). Nutraceutical use in late-stage cancer. *Cancer Metastasis Reviews*, 29(3), 503–510. Doi: 10.1007/s10555-010-9240-5.

7. Kundu, J.K., Na, H.K., Surh, Y.J. (2009). Ginger-derived phenolic substances with cancer preventive and therapeutic potential. *Forum of Nutrition*, 61, 182–192. Doi: 10.1159/000212750.

8. Lete, I., & Allué, J. (2016). The Effectiveness of Ginger in the Prevention of Nausea and Vomiting during

Pregnancy and Chemotherapy. *Integrative Medicine Insights*, 11, 11–17. Doi: 10.4137/IMI.S36273.

9. Rahnama, P., Montazeri, A., Huseini, H. F., Kianbakht, S., & Naseri, M. (2012). Effect of *Zingiber officinale* R. rhizomes (ginger) on pain relief in primary dysmenorrhea: a placebo randomized trial. *BMC Complementary and Alternative Medicine*, 12, 92. Doi: 10.1186/1472-6882-12-92.

10. Mashhadi, N. S., Ghiasvand, R., Askari, G., Hariri, M., Darvishi, L., & Mofid, M. R. (2013). Anti-Oxidative and Anti-Inflammatory Effects of Ginger in Health and Physical Activity: Review of Current Evidence. *International Journal of Preventive Medicine*, 4(Suppl 1), S36–S42.

11. Ibid, 10.

12. 1Heimes, K., Feistel, B., Verspohl, E.J. (2009). Impact of the 5-HT receptor channel system for insulin secretion and interaction of ginger extracts. *European Journal of Pharmacology*, 624, 58–65. Doi: 10.1016/j.ejphar.2009.09.049.

13. Sekiya K., Ohtani A., Kusano S. (2004). Enhancement of insulin sensitivity in adipocytes by ginger. *Biofactors*, 22, 153–6. https://www.ncbi.nlm.nih.gov/pubmed/15630272.

14. Ibid, 10.

15. Drobnic, F., Riera, J., Appendino, G., Togni, S., Franceschi, F., Valle, X., ... Tur, J. (2014). Reduction of delayed onset muscle soreness by a novel curcumin delivery system (Meriva®): a

randomised, placebo-controlled trial. *Journal of the International Society of Sports Nutrition*, 11, 31. Doi: 10.1186/1550-2783-11-31.

16. Karuppiah, P., & Rajaram, S. (2012). Antibacterial effect of *Allium sativum* cloves and *Zingiber officinale* rhizomes against multiple-drug resistant clinical pathogens. *Asian Pacific Journal of Tropical Biomedicine*, 2(8), 597–601. Doi:10.1016/S2221-1691(12)60104-X.

17. Rahman, S., Parvez, A. K., Islam, R., & Khan, M. H. (2011). Antibacterial activity of natural spices on multiple drug resistant Escherichia coli isolated from drinking water, Bangladesh. *Annals of Clinical Microbiology and Antimicrobials*, 10, 10. Doi: 10.1186/1476-0711-10-10.

18. Ibid, 17.

Chapter 14 – Turmeric

1. Prasad, S., Aggarwal, B, B. Turmeric, the Golden Spice: From Traditional Medicine to Modern Medicine. In: Benzie IFF, Wachtel-Galor S, editors. *Herbal Medicine: Biomolecular and Clinical Aspects* (2nd ed.). Boca Raton (FL): CRC Press/Taylor & Francis; 2011. Chapter 13. http://www.ncbi.nlm.nih.gov/books/NBK92752/ (accessed on May 11th, 2017).

2. Ibid, 1.

3. Agarwal, K.A., Tripathi, C.D., Agarwal, B.B., Saluja, S. (2011). Efficacy of turmeric (curcumin) in pain and postoperative fatigue after laparoscopic cholecystectomy: a double-blind, randomized placebo-controlled

study. *Surgical Endoscopy*, 25, 3805–10. Doi: 10.1007/s00464-011-1793-z.

4. Bundy, R., Walker, A.F., Middleton, R.W., Booth, J. (2004). Turmeric extract may improve irritable bowel syndrome symptomology in otherwise healthy adults: a pilot study. *The Journal of Alternative and Complementary Medicine*, 10, 1015–8. Doi: 10.1089/acm.2004.10.1015.

5. Kuptniratsaikul, V., Dajpratham, P., Taechaarpornkul, W., Buntragulpoontawee, M., Lukkanapichonchut, P., Chootip, C., Laongpech, S. (2014). Efficacy and safety of *Curcuma domestica* extracts compared with ibuprofen in patients with knee osteoarthritis: a multicenter study. *Clinical Interventions in Aging*, 9, 451–458. Doi: 10.2147/CIA.S58535.

6. Moghadam, A. R., Tutunchi, S., Namvaran-Abbas-Abad, A., Yazdi, M., Bonyadi, F., Mohajeri, D., Ghavami, S. (2015). Pre-administration of turmeric prevents methotrexate-induced liver toxicity and oxidative stress. *BMC Complementary and Alternative Medicine*, 15, 246. Doi: 10.1186/s12906-015-0773-6.

7. Gupta, S. C., Patchva, S., & Aggarwal, B. B. (2013). Therapeutic Roles of Curcumin: Lessons Learned from Clinical Trials. *The AAPS Journal*, 15(1), 195–218. Doi: 10.1208/s12248-012-9432-8.

8. Lin, L. I., Ke, Y. F., Ko, Y. C., Lin, J. K. (1998). Curcumin inhibits SK-hep-1 hepatocellular carcinoma cell invasion in vitro and suppresses matrix metalloproteinase-9 secretion. *Oncology*, 55, 349–353. Doi: 10.1159/000011876.

9. Haq, S., Ali, S., Mohammad, R., & Sarkar, F. H. (2012). The Complexities of Epidemiology and Prevention of Gastrointestinal Cancers. *International Journal of Molecular Sciences*, 13(10), 12556–12572. Doi: 10.3390/ijms131012556.

10. Chauhan, D.P. (2002). Chemotherapeutic potential of curcumin for colorectal cancer. *Current Pharmaceutical Design*, 8(19), 1695–1706. Doi: 10.2174/1381612023394016.

11. McCann, M. J., Johnston, S., Reilly, K., Men, X., Burgess, E. J., Perry, N. B., & Roy, N. C. (2014). The Effect of Turmeric (*Curcuma longa*) Extract on the Functionality of the Solute Carrier Protein 22 A4 (SLC22A4) and Interleukin-10 (IL-10) Variants Associated with Inflammatory Bowel Disease. *Nutrients*, 6(10), 4178–4190. Doi: 10.3390/nu6104178.

12. Aldini, R., Budriesi, R., Roda, G., Micucci, M., Ioan, P., D'Errico-Grigioni, A., Mazzella, G. (2012). *Curcuma longa* Extract Exerts a Myorelaxant Effect on the Ileum and Colon in a Mouse Experimental Colitis Model, Independent of the Anti-Inflammatory Effect. *PLoS ONE*, 7(9), e44650. Doi: 10.1371/journal.pone.0044650.

13. Aggarwal, B. B., & Harikumar, K. B. (2009). Potential Therapeutic Effects of Curcumin, the Anti-inflammatory Agent, Against Neurodegenerative, Cardiovascular, Pulmonary, Metabolic, Autoimmune and Neoplastic Diseases. *The International Journal of Biochemistry & Cell Biology*, 41(1), 40–59. Doi: 10.1016/j.biocel.2008.06.010.

14. Monsey, M. S., Gerhard, D. M., Boyle, L. M., Briones, M. A., Seligsohn, M., & Schafe, G. E. (2015). A Diet Enriched with Curcumin Impairs Newly Acquired and Reactivated Fear Memories. *Neuropsychopharmacology*, 40(5), 1278–1288. Doi: 10.1038/npp.2014.315.

15. Kulkarni, S., Dhir A., Akula, K .K. (2009). Potentials of curcumin as an antidepressant. *The Scientific World Journal*, 9, 1233–1241. Doi: 10.1100/tsw.2009.137.

16. 16. Khurana, S., Venkataraman, K., Hollingsworth, A., Piche, M., & Tai, T. C. (2013). Polyphenols: Benefits to the Cardiovascular System in Health and in Aging. *Nutrients*, 5(10), 3779–3827. Doi: 10.3390/nu5103779.

17. Moghadamtousi, S.Z., Kadir, H. A., Hassandarvish, P., Tajik, H., Abubakar, S., & Zandi, K. (2014). A Review on Antibacterial, Antiviral, and Antifungal Activity of Curcumin. *BioMed Research International*, 2014, 186864. Doi: 10.1155/2014/186864.

18. Ibid, 17.

19. Chen D-Y, Shien J-H, Tiley L., et al. (2010). Curcumin inhibits influenza virus infection and haemagglutination activity. *Food Chemistry*, 2010, 119(4), 1346–1351.

20. Upendra R.S., Khandelwal, P., Reddy A.H.M. (2011). Turmeric powder (*Curcuma longa Linn.*) as an antifungal agent in plant tissue culture studies. *International Journal of Engineering Science*, 3(11), 7899–7904.

21. Ibid, 13.

22. U.S. Food and Drug Administration (2018). CFR-Code of Federal Regulations Title 21 https://

www.accessdata.fda.gov/scripts/cdrh/cfdocs/cfcfr/
CFRSearch.cfm?fr=182.20

23. Lao, C. D., Ruffin, M. T., Normolle, D., Heath, D.
D., Murray, S. I., Bailey, J. M., Brenner, D. E. (2006).
Dose escalation of a curcuminoid formulation. *BMC
Complementary and Alternative Medicine*, 6, 10. Doi:
10.1186/1472-6882-6-10.

Chapter 15 - Cayenne

1. Whiting S., Derbyshire E., Tiwari, B.K. (2012).
Capsaicinoids and capsinoids. A potential role for
weight management? A systematic review of the
evidence. *Appetite*, 59(2), 341–348. Doi: 10.1016/j.
appet.2012.05.015.

2. Ibid, 1.

3. Sogut, O., Kaya, H., Gokdemir, M. T., & Sezen, Y.
(2012). Acute myocardial infarction and coronary vaso-
spasm associated with the ingestion of cayenne pepper
pills in a 25-year-old male. *International Journal of
Emergency Medicine*, 5, 5. Doi: 10.1186/1865-1380-5-5.

4. Kawabata. F., Inoue, N., Yazawa, S., Kawada, T., Inoue,
K., Fushiki, T. (2006). Effects of CH-19 sweet, a
non-pungent cultivar of red pepper, in decreasing the
body weight and suppressing body fat accumulation
by sympathetic nerve activation in humans. *Bioscience,
Biotechnology, and Biochemistry*, 70(12), 2824–2835.
Doi: 10.1271/bbb.60206.

5. Luo, X.J., Peng, J., Li, Y.J. (2011). Recent advances in
the study on capsaicinoids and capsinoids. *European*

Journal of Pharmacology, 650(1), 1–7. Doi: 10.1016/j.ejphar.2010.09.074.

6. Ibid, 5.

7. Wargovich, M. J., Morris, J., Brown, V., Ellis, J., Logothetis, B., & Weber, R. (2010). Nutraceutical use in late-stage cancer. *Cancer Metastasis Reviews*, 29(3), 503–510. Doi: 10.1007/s10555-010-9240-5.

Chapter 16 - Lemons

1. Kawaii, S., Tomono, Y., Katase, E., Ogawa, K., Yano, M., Koizumi M., et al. (2000). Quantitative study of flavonoids in leaves of Citrus plants. *Journal of Agricultural and Food Chemistry*, 48, 3865–71.

2. Raimondo, S., Naselli, F., Fontana, S., Monteleone, F., Lo Dico, A., Saieva, L., ... Alessandro, R. (2015). *Citrus limon*-derived nanovesicles inhibit cancer cell proliferation and suppress CML xenograft growth by inducing TRAIL-mediated cell death. *Oncotarget*, 6(23), 19514–19527.

3. Gualdani, R., Cavalluzzi, M.M., Lentini, G., Habtemariam, S. (2016). The Chemistry and Pharmacology of Citrus Limonoids. *Molecules*, 21(11),1530.

4. Bae, J-M., & Kim, E. H. (2016). Dietary intakes of citrus fruit and risk of gastric cancer incidence: an adaptive meta-analysis of cohort studies. *Epidemiology and Health*, 38, e2016034. Doi: 10.4178/epih.e2016034.

5. Ibid, 2.

6. Gamboa-Gómez, C. I., Rocha-Guzmán, N. E., Gallegos-Infante, J. A., Moreno-Jiménez, M. R., Vázquez-Cabral, B. D., & González-Laredo, R. F. (2015). Plants with potential use on obesity and its complications. *EXCLI Journal*, 14, 809–831. Doi: 10.17179/excli2015-186.

7. Fukuchi, Y., Hiramitsu, M., Okada, M., Hayashi, S., Nabeno, Y., Osawa, T., & Naito, M. (2008). Lemon Polyphenols Suppress Diet-induced Obesity by Up-Regulation of mRNA Levels of the Enzymes Involved in ß-Oxidation in Mouse White Adipose Tissue. *Journal of Clinical Biochemistry and Nutrition*, 43(3), 201–209. Doi: 10.3164/jcbn.2008066.

Chapter 17 - Garlic

1. Hatfield, G. (2004). *Encyclopedia of folk medicine: Old world and new world traditions.* Santa Barbara, Calif: ABC-CLIO.

2. Lin, P.-H., Aronson, W., & Freedland, S. J. (2015). Nutrition, dietary interventions and prostate cancer: the latest evidence. *BMC Medicine*, 13, 3. Doi: 10.1186/s12916-014-0234-y.

3. Hsing, A.W., Chokkalingam, A.P., Gao, Y.T., et al. (2002). Allium vegetables and risk of prostate cancer: A population-based study. *Journal of the National Cancer Institute*, 94(21), 1648–1651.

4. Gao, C.M., Takezaki, T., Ding, J.H., Li, M.S., Tajima, K. (1999). Protective effect of allium vegetables against both esophageal and stomach cancer: a simultaneous case-referent study of a high-epidemic area in Jiangsu

Province, China. *Japanese Journal of Cancer Research*, 90, 614–621.

5. Setiawan, V. W., Yu, G.-P., Lu, Q.-Y., Lu, M.-L., Yu, S.-Z., Mu, L., Zhang, Z.-F. (2005). Allium Vegetables and Stomach Cancer Risk in China. *Asian Pacific Journal of Cancer Prevention*, 6(3), 387–395.

6. Jin, Z.-Y., Wu, M., Han, R.-Q., Zhang, X.-F., Wang, X.-S., Liu, A.-M., Zhao, J.-K. (2013). Raw garlic consumption as a protective factor for lung cancer, a population-based case-control study in a Chinese population. *American Association of Cancer Research, Cancer Prevention Research (Philadelphia, Pa.)*, 6(7), 711–718. Doi: 10.1158/1940-6207.CAPR-13-0015.

7. Zhang, H., Wang, K., Lin, G., & Zhao, Z. (2014). Antitumor mechanisms of S-allyl mercaptocysteine for breast cancer therapy. *BMC Complementary and Alternative Medicine*, 14, 270. Doi: 10.1186/1472-6882-14-270.

8. Antony, M. L., & Singh, S. V. (2011). Molecular Mechanisms and Targets of Cancer Chemoprevention by Garlic-derived Bioactive Compound Diallyl Trisulfide. *Indian Journal of Experimental Biology*, 49(11), 805–816.

9. Herman-Antosiewicz A., Singh, S.V. (2004). Signal transduction pathways leading to cell cycle arrest and apoptosis induction in cancer cells by Allium vegetable-derived organosulfur compounds: a review. *Mutation research*, 555, 121–31.

10. Milner J.A. (2001). A historical perspective on garlic and cancer. *The Journal of nutrition*, 131, 1027S–31S.

11. Nicastro, H. L., Ross, S. A., & Milner, J. A. (2015). Garlic and onions: Their cancer prevention properties. *Cancer Prevention Research (Philadelphia, Pa.)*, 8(3), 181–189. Doi: 10.1158/1940-6207.CAPR-14-0172.

12. National Cancer Institute (2017). Garlic and Cancer Prevention. https://www.cancer.gov/about-cancer/causes-prevention/risk/diet/garlic-fact-sheet (accessed on May 11th, 2017).

13. Adetumbi, M.A., Lau, B.H. (1983). Allium sativum (garlic)--a natural antibiotic. *Medical hypotheses*, 12, 227–37.

Chapter 18 - Cloves

1. Wikipedia (2017). The Free Encyclopedia. Clove. https://en.wikipedia.org/wiki/Clove (accessed on May 11th, 2017)

2. Kumar, P. S., Febriyanti, R. M., Sofyan, F. F., Luftimas, D. E., & Abdulah, R. (2014). Anticancer potential of *Syzygium aromaticum L.* in MCF-7 human breast cancer cell lines. *Pharmacognosy Research*, 6(4), 350–354. Doi: 10.4103/0974-8490.138291.

3. Ibid, 2.

4. Liu, H., Schmitz, J. C., Wei, J., Cao, S., Beumer, J. H., Strychor, S., Lin, X. (2014). Clove Extract Inhibits Tumor Growth and Promotes Cell Cycle Arrest and Apoptosis. *Oncology Research*, 21(5), 247–259. Doi: 10.3727/096504014X13946388748910.

5. Ibid, 4.

6. Al-Sharif, I., Remmal, A., & Aboussekhra, A. (2013). Eugenol triggers apoptosis in breast cancer cells through E2F1/survivin down-regulation. *BMC Cancer*, 13, 600. Doi: 10.1186/1471-2407-13-600.

7. Ali, S., Prasad, R., Mahmood, A., Routray, I., Shinkafi, T. S., Sahin, K., & Kucuk, O. (2014). Eugenol-rich Fraction of *Syzygium aromaticum* (Clove) Reverses Biochemical and Histopathological Changes in Liver Cirrhosis and Inhibits Hepatic Cell Proliferation. *Journal of Cancer Prevention*, 19(4), 288–300. Doi: 10.15430/JCP.2014.19.4.288.

8. Ahmad, T., Shinkafi, T. S., Routray, I., Mahmood, A., & Ali, S. (2012). Aqueous Extract of Dried Flower Buds of *Syzygium aromaticum* Inhibits Inflammation and Oxidative Stress. *Journal of Basic and Clinical Pharmacy*, 3(3), 323–327.

9. Khan, A., Qadir, S.S., Khattak, K.N., & Anderson, R. (2006). Cloves improve glucose, cholesterol and triglycerides of people with type 2 diabetes mellitus. *The Federation of American Societies for Experimental Biology*, 20, A990.

10. Ibid, 9.

11. Sompong, W., Muangngam, N., Kongpatpharnich, A., Manacharoenlarp, C., Amorworasin, C., Suantawee, T., Adisakwattana, S. (2016). The inhibitory activity of herbal medicines on the keys enzymes and steps related to carbohydrate and lipid digestion. *BMC Complementary and Alternative Medicine*, 16, 439. Doi: 10.1186/s12906-016-1424-2.

12. Ibid, 11.

13. The U.S. Food & Drug Administration (2017). Select Committee on GRAS Substances (SCOGS) Opinion: Clove Bud Extract, Clove Bud Oil, Clove Bud Oleoresin, Clove Leaf Oil, Clove Stem Oil, Eugenol. http://www.fda.gov/Food/IngredientsPackagingLabeling/GRAS/SCOGS/ucm261254.htm (accessed on May 11th, 2017).

14. The U. S. National Library of Medicine. Medline Plus (2017). Clove. https://medlineplus.gov/druginfo/natural/251.html (accessed on May 11th, 2017).

15. Ibid,14.

16. Ibid, 14.

Chapter 19 - Cinnamon

1. WebMD (2017). Cinnamon. http://www.webmd.com/diet/supplement-guide-cinnamon (accessed on May 11th, 2017).

2. Ibid, 1.

3. Ibid, 1.

4. Miller, K. G., Poole, C. F. and Chichila, T. M. P. (1995), Solvent-assisted supercritical fluid extraction for the isolation of semi volatile flavor compounds from the cinnamons of commerce and their separation by series-coupled column gas chromatography. *Journal of Separation Science*, 18(8), 461–510. Doi: 10.1002/jhrc.1240180802.

5. Wijesekera, R.O. (1978). Historical overview of the cinnamon industry. *CRC Critical Reviews in Food Science and Nutrition*, 10, 1–30.

6. National Center for Biotechnology Information (2017). *Cinnamomum verum.* https://www.ncbi.nlm.nih.gov/Taxonomy/Browser/wwwtax.cgi?id=128608 (accessed on May 11th, 2017).

7. Ranasinghe, P., Pigera, S., Premakumara, G. S., Galappaththy, P., Constantine, G. R., & Katulanda, P. (2013). Medicinal properties of "true" cinnamon (*Cinnamomum zeylanicum*): a systematic review. *BMC Complementary and Alternative Medicine*, 13, 275. Doi: 10.1186/1472-6882-13-275.

8. Ibid, 7.

9. Lu, T., Sheng, H., Wu, J., Cheng, Y., Zhu, J., Chen, Y. (2012). Cinnamon extract improves fasting blood glucose and glycosylated hemoglobin level in Chinese patients with type 2 diabetes *Nutrition Research*, 32(6), 408-412.

10. Ranasinghe, P., Perera, S., Gunatilake, M., Abeywardene, E., Gunapala, N., Premakumara, S., Katulanda, P. (2012). Effects of *Cinnamomum zeylanicum* (Ceylon cinnamon) on blood glucose and lipids in a diabetic and healthy rat model. *Pharmacognosy Research*, 4(2), 73–79. Doi: 10.4103/0974-8490.94719.

11. Sartorius, T., Peter, A., Schulz, N., Drescher, A., Bergheim, I., Machann, J., Hennige, A. M. (2014). Cinnamon Extract Improves Insulin Sensitivity in the Brain and Lowers Liver Fat in Mouse Models of Obesity. *PLoS ONE*, 9(3), e92358. Doi: 10.1371/journal.pone.0092358.

12. Ibid, 11.

13. Allen, R. W., Schwartzman, E., Baker, W. L., Coleman, C. I., & Phung, O. J. (2013). Cinnamon Use in Type 2 Diabetes: An Updated Systematic Review and Meta-Analysis. *Annals of Family Medicine*, 11(5), 452–459. Doi: 10.1370/afm.1517.

14. Ibid, 13.

15. Anderson, R. A., Qin, B., Canini, F., Poulet, L., & Roussel, A. M. (2013). Cinnamon Counteracts the Negative Effects of a High Fat/High Fructose Diet on Behavior, Brain Insulin Signaling and Alzheimer-Associated Changes. *PLoS ONE*, 8(12), e83243. Doi: 10.1371/journal.pone.0083243.

16. Ibid, 15.

17. Kwon, H.K., Jeon, W.K., Hwang, J.S., Lee, C.G., So, J.S., Park, J.A., et al. (2009). Cinnamon extract suppresses tumor progression by modulating angiogenesis and the effector function of CD8+ T cells. *Cancer Letters*, 278, 174–82.

18. Kwon, H.-K., Hwang, J.-S., So, J.-S., Lee, C.-G., Sahoo, A., Ryu, J.-H., Im, S.-H. (2010). Cinnamon extract induces tumor cell death through inhibition of NFkB and AP1. *BMC Cancer*, 10, 392. Doi: 10.1186/1471-2407-10-392.

19. Ibid, 17.

20. Ibid, 7.

21. Nyadjeu, P., Nguelefack-Mbuyo, E. P., Atsamo, A. D., Nguelefack, T. B., Dongmo, A. B., & Kamanyi, A. (2013). Acute and chronic antihypertensive effects of *Cinnamomum zeylanicum* stem bark methanol

extract in L-NAME-induced hypertensive rats. *BMC Complementary and Alternative Medicine*, 13, 27. Doi: 10.1186/1472-6882-13-27.

22. Ibid, 7.

23. Dhuley, J.N. (1999). Anti-oxidant effects of cinnamon (*Cinnamomum verum*) bark and greater cardamon (*Amomum subulatum*) seeds in rats fed high fat diet. *Indian Journal of Experimental Biology*, 37(3), 238–242.

Chapter 20 - The Mint Family

Rosemary

1. Encyclopedia Britannica (2017). Lamiaceae Plant Family. https://www.britannica.com/plant/Lamiaceae (accessed on May 11th, 2017).

2. Rousseau, B. (2016, October 19). What In The World. Rosemary and Time: Does This Italian Hamlet Have a Recipe for Long Life? The New York Times. https://www.nytimes.com/2016/10/20/world/what-in-the-world/rosemary-and-time-does-this-italian-hamlet-have-a-recipe-for-long-life.html?_r=1 (accessed on May 11th, 2017)

3. Ibid, 2.

4. Ibid, 2.

5. Borrás-Linares, I., Stojanovic, Z., Quirantes-Piné, R., Arráez-Román, D., Švarc-Gajic, J., Fernández-Gutiérrez, A., & Segura-Carretero, A. (2014). *Rosmarinus Officinalis* Leaves as a Natural Source of Bioactive Compounds. *International Journal of*

Molecular Sciences, 15(11), 20585–20606. Doi: 10.3390/ ijms151120585.

6. Ibid, 5.

7. Ibid, 5.

8. De Oliveira, M.R. (2016). The Dietary Components Carnosic Acid and Carnosol as Neuroprotective Agents: a Mechanistic View. *Molecular Neurobiology*, 53(9), 6155-6168.

9. Ibid, 5.

10. Ibid, 8.

11. Kim S., Kim, J., Cho, H., Lee, H.J., Kim, S.Y., Kim, S., Lee S., Chun, H.S. (2006). Carnosol, a component of rosemary (*Rosmarinus officinalis L.*) protects nigral dopaminergic neuronal cells. *Neuroreport*, 17, 1729–1733. Doi: 10.1097/01.wnr.0000239951.14954.10.

12. Habtemariam, S. (2016). The Therapeutic Potential of Rosemary (*Rosmarinus officinalis*) Diterpenes for Alzheimer's Disease. Evidence-Based Complementary and Alternative Medicine, article ID, 2680409. Doi: 10.1155/2016/2680409.

13. Ibid, 12.

14. Ibid, 2.

15. Ibid, 2.

16. Bermejo, L.M., López-Plaza, B., Weber, T.K., Palma-Milla, S., Iglesias, C., Reglero, G., Gómez-Candela, C. (2014). Impact of cooked functional meat enriched with omega-3 fatty acids and rosemary extract on

inflammatory and oxidative status; a randomised, double-blind, crossover study. *Nutricion Hospitalaria*, 30(5), 1084-91. Doi: 10.3305/nh.2014.30.5.8048.

17. Puangsombat, K., Smith, J.S. (2010). Inhibition of heterocyclic amine formation in beef patties by ethanolic extracts of rosemary. *Journal of Food Science*, 75, T40–T47. Doi: 10.1111/j.1750-3841.2009.01491.x.

18. Sayorwan, W., Ruangrungsi, N., Piriyapunyporn, T., Hongratanaworakit, T., Kotchabhakdi, N., & Siripornpanich, V. (2013). Effects of Inhaled Rosemary Oil on Subjective Feelings and Activities of the Nervous System. *Scientia Pharmaceutica*, 81(2), 531–542. Doi: 10.3797/scipharm.1209-05.

19. Organisciak, D. T., Darrow, R. M., Rapp, C. M., Smuts, J. P., Armstrong, D. W., & Lang, J. C. (2013). Prevention of retinal light damage by zinc oxide combined with rosemary extract. *Molecular Vision*, 19, 1433–1445.

20. Moore, J., Yousef, M., & Tsiani, E. (2016). Anticancer Effects of Rosemary (*Rosmarinus officinalis L.*) Extract and Rosemary Extract Polyphenols. *Nutrients*, 8(11), 731. Doi: 10.3390/nu8110731.

Thyme

1. Hossain, M. A., AL-Raqmi, K. A. S., AL-Mijizy, Z. H., Weli, A. M., & Al-Riyami, Q. (2013). Study of total phenol, flavonoids contents and phytochemical screening of various leaves crude extracts of locally grown *Thymus vulgaris*. *Asian Pacific Journal of Tropical Biomedicine*, 3(9), 705–710. Doi: 10.1016/S2221-1691(13)60142-2.

2. Palaniappan, K., Holley, R.A. (2010). Use of natural antimicrobials to increase antibiotic susceptibility of drug resistant bacteria. *International Journal of Food Microbiology*, 140(2), 164-168. Doi: 10.1016/j.ijfoodmicro.2010.04.001.

3. Boruga, O., Jianu, C., Misca, C., Golet, I., Gruia, A., & Horhat, F. (2014). *Thymus vulgaris* essential oil: chemical composition and antimicrobial activity. *Journal of Medicine and Life*, 7(Spec Iss 3), 56–60.

4. Ibid, 3.

5. Salmalian, H., Saghebi, R., Moghadamnia, A. A., Bijani, A., Faramarzi, M., Nasiri Amiri, F., Bekhradi, R. (2014). Comparative effect of *thymus vulgaris* and ibuprofen on primary dysmenorrhea: A triple-blind clinical study. *Caspian Journal of Internal Medicine*, 5(2), 82–88.

6. Mihailovic-Stanojevic, N., Miloradovic, Z., Ivanov, M., Bugarski, B., Jovovic, Đ., Karanovic, D., Grujic-Milanovic, J. (2016). Upregulation of Heme Oxygenase-1 in Response to Wild Thyme Treatment Protects against Hypertension and Oxidative Stress. *Oxidative Medicine and Cellular Longevity*, 1458793. Doi: 10.1155/2016/1458793.

7. Ibid, 3.

8. Shimelis, N. D., Asticcioli, S., Baraldo, M., Tirillini, B., Lulekal, E. and Murgia, V. (2012), Researching accessible and affordable treatment for common dermatological problems in developing countries. An Ethiopian experience. *International Journal of Dermatology*, 51, 790–795. Doi: 10.1111/j.1365-4632.2011.05235.x

Oregano

1. Coccimiglio, J., Alipour, M., Jiang, Z.-H., Gottardo, C., & Suntres, Z. (2016). Antioxidant, Antibacterial, and Cytotoxic Activities of the Ethanolic *Origanum vulgare* Extract and Its Major Constituents. *Oxidative Medicine and Cellular Longevity*, 2016, 1404505. Doi: 10.1155/2016/1404505.

2. Li, Z., Henning, S. M., Zhang, Y., Zerlin, A., Li, L., Gao, K., Heber, D. (2010). Antioxidant-rich spice added to hamburger meat during cooking results in reduced meat, plasma, and urine malondialdehyde concentrations. *The American Journal of Clinical Nutrition*, 91(5), 1180–1184. Doi: 10.3945/ajcn.2009.28526.

3. Ibid, 2.

4. 4. Henning S. M., Zhang Y., Seeram N. P., et al. (2011). Antioxidant capacity and phytochemical content of herbs and spices in dry, fresh and blended herb paste form. *International Journal of Food Sciences and Nutrition*, 62(3):219–225. Doi: 10.3109/09637486.2010.530595.

5. Ibid, 4.

6. Ibid, 4.

7. Ben-Arye, E., Dudai, N., Eini, A., Torem, M., Schiff, E., & Rakover, Y. (2011). Treatment of Upper Respiratory Tract Infections in Primary Care: A Randomized Study Using Aromatic Herbs. *Evidence-Based Complementary and Alternative Medicine*, 2011, 690346. Doi: 10.1155/2011/690346.

8. Ibid, 1.

Chapter 21 - Teas from Your Kitchen

Green Tea

1. Forester, S. C., & Lambert, J. D. (2011). Antioxidant effects of green tea. *Molecular Nutrition & Food Research*, 55(6), 844–854. Doi: 10.1002/mnfr.201000641.

2. Lin, Y.S., Tsai, Y.J., Tsay, J.S., Lin, J.K. (2003). Factors affecting the levels of tea polyphenols and caffeine in tea leaves. *Journal of Agricultural and Food Chemistry*, 51(7), 1864–1873. Doi: 10.1021/jf021066b.

3. Li, Z., Henning, S. M., Zhang, Y., Zerlin, A., Li, L., Gao, K., Heber, D. (2010). Antioxidant-rich spice added to hamburger meat during cooking results in reduced meat, plasma, and urine malondialdehyde concentrations. *The American Journal of Clinical Nutrition*, 91(5), 1180–1184. Doi: 10.3945/ajcn.2009.28526.

4. Tsai, Y.-J., & Chen, B.-H. (2016). Preparation of catechin extracts and nanoemulsions from green tea leaf waste and their inhibition effect on prostate cancer cell PC-3. *International Journal of Nanomedicine*, 11, 1907–1926. Doi: 10.2147/IJN.S103759.

5. Cavet, M. E., Harrington, K. L., Vollmer, T. R., Ward, K. W., & Zhang, J.-Z. (2011). Anti-inflammatory and anti-oxidative effects of the green tea polyphenol epigallocatechin gallate in human corneal epithelial cells. *Molecular Vision*, 17, 533–542.

6. Kang, K. S., Yamabe, N., Wen, Y., Fukui, M., & Zhu, B. T. (2013). Beneficial Effects of Natural Phenolics on Levodopa Methylation and Oxidative

Neurodegeneration. *Brain Research*, 1497, 1–14. Doi: 10.1016/j.brainres.2012.11.043.

7. Ibid, 6.

8. Ibid, 1.

9. Lamothe, S., Azimy, N., Bazinet, L., Couillard, C., Britten, M. (2014). Interaction of green tea polyphenols with dairy matrices in a simulated gastrointestinal environment. *Food & Function*, 5, 2621–2631. Doi: 10.1039/C4FO00203B.

Mint

1. Londonkar, R. L., & Poddar, P. V. (2009). Studies on activity of various extracts of *Mentha arvensis Linn* against drug induced gastric ulcer in mammals. *World Journal of Gastrointestinal Oncology*, 1(1), 82–88. Doi: 10.4251/wjgo.v1.i1.82.

2. Liu, X., Sun, Z.-L., Jia, A.-R., Shi, Y.-P., Li, R.-H., & Yang, P.-M. (2014). Extraction, Preliminary Characterization and Evaluation of in Vitro Antitumor and Antioxidant Activities of Polysaccharides from *Mentha piperita*. *International Journal of Molecular Sciences*, 15(9), 16302–16319. Doi: 10.3390/ijms150916302.

3. Al-Bayati, F. A. (2009). Isolation and identification of antimicrobial compound from *Mentha longifolia L.* leaves grown wild in Iraq. *Annals of Clinical Microbiology and Antimicrobials*, 8, 20. Doi: 10.1186/1476-0711-8-20.

4. Inoue, T., Sugimoto, Y., Masuda, H., Kamei, C. (2002). Antiallergic effect of flavonoid glycosides obtained

from *Mentha piperita L. Biological and Pharmaceutical Bulletin*, 25, 256–259. Doi: 10.1248/bpb.25.256.

5. Jaradat, N. A., Al Zabadi, H., Rahhal, B., Hussein, A. M. A., Mahmoud, J. S., Mansour, B., Issa, A. (2016). The effect of inhalation of *Citrus sinensis* flowers and *Mentha spicata* leave essential oils on lung function and exercise performance: a quasi-experimental uncontrolled before-and-after study. Journal of the International Society of Sports Nutrition, 13, 36. Doi: 10.1186/s12970-016-0146-7.

6. Ibid, 5.

7. Ibid, 2.

8. Oh, J. Y., Park, M. A., & Kim, Y. C. (2014). Peppermint Oil Promotes Hair Growth without Toxic Signs. *Toxicological Research*, 30(4), 297–304. Doi: 10.5487/TR.2014.30.4.297.

Chapter 22 - Superfoods In Review

Kaempferol

1. Encyclopedia Wikipedia. Kaempferol. https://en.wikipedia.org/wiki/Kaempferol (accessed on May 11th, 2017).

2. Chen, A. Y., & Chen, Y. C. (2013). A review of the dietary flavonoid, kaempferol on human health and cancer chemoprevention. *Food Chemistry*, 138(4), 2099–2107. Doi: 10.1016/j.foodchem.2012.11.139.

3. Ibid, 2.

4. Ibid, 2.

5. Alkhalidy, H., Moore, W., Zhang, Y., McMillan, R., Wang, A., Ali, M., Liu, D. (2015). Small Molecule Kaempferol Promotes Insulin Sensitivity and Preserved Pancreatic ß-Cell Mass in Middle-Aged Obese Diabetic Mice. *Journal of Diabetes Research*, 2015, 532984. Doi: 10.1155/2015/532984.

6. Ibid, 5.

7. Park, S., Sapkota, K., Kim, S., Kim, H., & Kim, S. (2011). Kaempferol acts through mitogen-activated protein kinases and protein kinase B/AKT to elicit protection in a model of neuroinflammation in BV2 microglial cells. *British Journal of Pharmacology*, 164(3), 1008–1025. Doi: 10.1111/j.1476-5381.2011.01389.x.

8. Kim, I.-R., Kim, S.-E., Baek, H.-S., Kim, B.-J., Kim, C.-H., Chung, I.-K., Shin, S.-H. (2016). The role of kaempferol-induced autophagy on differentiation and mineralization of osteoblastic MC3T3-E1 cells. *BMC Complementary and Alternative Medicine*, 16(1), 333. Doi: 10.1186/s12906-016-1320-9.

9. Li, Y., Ding, Z., & Wu, C. (2016). Mechanistic Study of the Inhibitory Effect of Kaempferol on Uterine Fibroids In Vitro. Medical Science Monitor. *International Medical Journal of Experimental and Clinical Research*, 22, 4803–4808. Doi: 10.12659/MSM.898127.

10. Ibid, 9.

11. Zhou, M., Ren, H., Han, J., Wang, W., Zheng, Q., & Wang, D. (2015). Protective Effects of Kaempferol against Myocardial Ischemia/Reperfusion Injury in Isolated Rat Heart via Antioxidant Activity and

Inhibition of Glycogen Synthase Kinase-3ß. *Oxidative Medicine and Cellular Longevity*, 2015, 481405. Doi: 10.1155/2015/481405.

Luteolin

1. Ibid, Chapter 19, # 4.

2. Pratheeshkumar, P., Son, Y.-O., Budhraja, A., Wang, X., Ding, S., Wang, L., Shi, X. (2012). Luteolin Inhibits Human Prostate Tumor Growth by Suppressing Vascular Endothelial Growth Factor Receptor 2-Mediated Angiogenesis. *PLoS ONE*, 7(12), e52279. Doi: 10.1371/journal.pone.0052279.

3. Ibid, 2.

4. Cheng, W.-Y., Chiao, M.-T., Liang, Y.-J., Yang, Y.-C., Shen, C.-C., & Yang, C.-Y. (2013). Luteolin inhibits migration of human glioblastoma U-87 MG and T98G cells through downregulation of Cdc42 expression and PI3K/AKT activity. *Molecular Biology Reports*, 40(9), 5315–5326. Doi: 10.1007/s11033-013-2632-1.

5. Lin, Y., Shi, R., Wang, X., & Shen, H.-M. (2008). Luteolin, a flavonoid with potentials for cancer prevention and therapy. *Current Cancer Drug Targets*, 8(7), 634–646.

6. Ibid, 5.

7. Li, M., Li, Q., Zhao, Q., Zhang, J., & Lin, J. (2015). Luteolin improves the impaired nerve functions in diabetic neuropathy: behavioral and biochemical evidences. *International Journal of Clinical and Experimental Pathology*, 8(9), 10112–10120.

8. Sun, D., Huang, J., Zhang, Z., Gao, H., Li, J., Shen, M., Wang, H. (2012). Luteolin Limits Infarct Size and Improves Cardiac Function after Myocardium Ischemia/Reperfusion Injury in Diabetic Rats. *PLoS ONE*, 7(3), e33491. Doi: 10.1371/journal. pone.0033491.

9. Wu, X., Xu, T., Li, D., Zhu, S., Chen, Q., Hu, W., Sun, H. (2013). ERK/PP1a/PLB/SERCA2a and JNK Pathways Are Involved in Luteolin-Mediated Protection of Rat Hearts and Cardiomyocytes following Ischemia/Reperfusion. *PLoS ONE*, 8(12), e82957. Doi: 10.1371/journal.pone.0082957.

10. Xia, N., Chen, G., Liu, M., Ye, X., Pan, Y., Ge, J., Xie, S. (2016). Anti-inflammatory effects of luteolin on experimental autoimmune thyroiditis in mice. *Experimental and Therapeutic Medicine*, 12(6), 4049–4054. Doi: 10.3892/etm.2016.3854.

Myricetin

1. Semwal, D. K., Semwal, R. B., Combrinck, S., & Viljoen, A. (2016). Myricetin: A Dietary Molecule with Diverse Biological Activities. *Nutrients*, 8(2), 90. Doi: 10.3390/nu8020090.

2. Bennett C. J., Caldwell S.T., McPhail D.B., Morrice P.C., Duthie G.G., Hartley R.C. (2004). Potential therapeutic antioxidants that combine the radical scavenging ability of myricetin and the lipophilic chain of vitamin E to effectively inhibit microsomal lipid peroxidation. *Bioorganic & Medicinal Chemistry*, 12, 2079–2098. Doi: 10.1016/j.bmc.2004.02.031. https:// www.ncbi.nlm.nih.gov/pubmed/15080911.

3. Su, H., Feng, L., Zheng, X., & Chen, W. (2016). Myricetin protects against diet-induced obesity and ameliorates oxidative stress in C57BL/6 mice . *Journal of Zhejiang University. Science. B*, 17(6), 437–446. Doi: 10.1631/jzus.B1600074.

4. Ibid, 3.

5. Ibid, 1.

6. Huang, H., Chen, A. Y., Ye, X., Li, B., Rojanasakul, Y., Rankin, G. O., & Chen, Y. C. (2015). Myricetin inhibits proliferation of cisplatin-resistant cancer cells through a p53-dependent apoptotic pathway. *International Journal of Oncology*, 47(4), 1494–1502. Doi: 10.3892/ijo.2015.3133.

7. Zhang, S., Wang, L., Liu, H., Zhao, G., & Ming, L. (2014). Enhancement of recombinant myricetin on the radiosensitivity of lung cancer A549 and H1299 cells. *Diagnostic Pathology*, 9, 68. Doi: 10.1186/1746-1596-9-68.

Quercetin

1. Li, Y., Yao, J., Han, C., Yang, J., Chaudhry, M. T., Wang, S., ... Yin, Y. (2016). Quercetin, Inflammation and Immunity. *Nutrients*, 8(3), 167. Doi: 10.3390/nu8030167.

2. Ibid, 1.

3. Ibid, 1.

4. Brüll, V., Burak, C., Stoffel-Wagner, B., Wolffram, S., Nickenig, G., Müller, C., Egert, S. (2015). Effects of a quercetin-rich onion skin extract on 24 h ambulatory

blood pressure and endothelial function in overweight-to-obese patients with (pre-)hypertension: a randomised double-blinded placebo-controlled cross-over trial. *The British Journal of Nutrition*, 114(8), 1263–1277. Doi: 10.1017/S0007114515002950.

5. Brüll V., Burak C., Stoffel-Wagner B., Wolffram S., Nickenig G., Muller C., ... Egert, S. (2017). Acute intake of quercetin from onion skin extract does not influence postprandial blood pressure and endothelial function in overweight-to-obese adults with hypertension: a randomized, double-blind, placebo-controlled, crossover trial. *European Journal of Nutrition*, 56(3), 1347-1357. Doi: 10.1007/s00394-016-1185-1.

6. Khurana, S., Venkataraman, K., Hollingsworth, A., Piche, M., & Tai, T. C. (2013). Polyphenols: Benefits to the Cardiovascular System in Health and in Aging. *Nutrients*, 5(10), 3779–3827. Doi: 10.3390/nu5103779.

7. Nekohashi, M., Ogawa, M., Ogihara, T., Nakazawa, K., Kato, H., Misaka, T., Kobayashi, S. (2014). Luteolin and Quercetin Affect the Cholesterol Absorption Mediated by Epithelial Cholesterol Transporter Niemann–Pick C1-Like 1 in Caco-2 Cells and Rats. *PLoS ONE*, 9(5), e97901. Doi: 10.1371/journal.pone.0097901.

8. Wu, W., Li, R., Li, X., He, J., Jiang, S., Liu, S., & Yang, J. (2016). Quercetin as an Antiviral Agent Inhibits Influenza A Virus (IAV) Entry. *Viruses*, 8(1), 6. Doi: 10.3390/v8010006.

9. Ko, C.-C., Chen, Y.-J., Chen, C.-T., Liu, Y.-C., Cheng, F.-C., Hsu, K.-C., & Chow, L.-P. (2014). Chemical Proteomics Identifies Heterogeneous Nuclear

Ribonucleoprotein (hnRNP) A1 as the Molecular Target of Quercetin in Its Anti-Cancer Effects in PC-3 Cells. *The Journal of Biological Chemistry*, 289(32), 22078–22089. Doi: 10.1074/jbc.M114.553248.

10. Ranganathan, S., Halagowder, D., & Sivasithambaram, N. D. (2015). Quercetin Suppresses Twist to Induce Apoptosis in MCF-7 Breast Cancer Cells. *PLoS ONE*, 10(10), e0141370. Doi: 10.1371/journal.pone.0141370.

11. Djuric, Z., Severson, R. K., & Kato, I. (2012). Association of Dietary Quercetin with Reduced Risk of Proximal Colon Cancer. *Nutrition and Cancer*, 64(3), 351–360. Doi: 10.1080/01635581.2012.658950.

Chapter 23 - The True Superheroes

1. Pérez-Cano, F. J., & Castell, M. (2016). Flavonoids, Inflammation and Immune System. *Nutrients*, 8(10), 659. Doi: 10.3390/nu8100659.

2. Zamora-Ros, R., Forouhi, N. G., Sharp, S. J., González, C. A., Buijsse, B., Guevara, M., Wareham, N. J. (2014). Dietary Intakes of Individual Flavanols and Flavonols Are Inversely Associated with Incident Type 2 Diabetes in European Populations. *The Journal of Nutrition*, 144(3), 335–343. Doi: 10.3945/jn.113.184945.

3. Cassidy, A., Huang, T., Rice, M. S., Rimm, E. B., & Tworoger, S. S. (2014). Intake of dietary flavonoids and risk of epithelial ovarian cancer. *The American Journal of Clinical Nutrition*, 100(5), 1344–1351. Doi: 10.3945/ajcn.114.088708.

4. Hua, X., Yu, L., You, R., Yang, Y., Liao, J., Chen, D., & Yu, L. (2016). Association among Dietary Flavonoids,

Flavonoid Subclasses and Ovarian Cancer Risk: A Meta-Analysis. *PLoS ONE*, 11(3), e0151134. Doi: 10.1371/journal.pone.0151134.

5. Ibid, 1.

Chapter 24 - Machines And Oils: Why The Body?

1. Encyclopedia Wikipedia. Smoke Point. https://en.wikipedia.org/wiki/Smoke_point on (accessed on May 11th, 2017).

2. Harvard School of Public Health (2017). Eating fried foods tied to increased risk of diabetes, heart disease. https://www.hsph.harvard.edu/news/hsph-in-the-news/eating-fried-foods-tied-to-increased-risk-of-diabetes-and-heart-disease/ (accessed on May 11th, 2017).

3. Ibid, 2.

Chapter 25 - Mix Right, Further The Boost

1. Hossein-nezhad, A., & Holick, M. F. (2013). Vitamin D for Health: A Global Perspective. Mayo Clinic Proceedings. *Mayo Clinic*, 88(7), 720–755. Doi: 10.1016/j.mayocp.2013.05.011.

2. Sabinsa Corporation (2017). BioPerine. http://www.sabinsa.com/products/standardized-phytoextracts/bioperine/ (accessed on May 11th, 2017).

3. Li, Z., Henning, S. M., Zhang, Y., Zerlin, A., Li, L., Gao, K., Heber, D. (2010). Antioxidant-rich spice added to hamburger meat during cooking results in reduced meat, plasma, and urine malondialdehyde

concentrations. *The American Journal of Clinical Nutrition*, 91(5), 1180–1184. Doi: 10.3945/ajcn.2009.28526.

4. Ibid, 3.

5. Xiong, J. S., Branigan, D., & Li, M. (2009). Deciphering the MSG controversy. *International Journal of Clinical and Experimental Medicine*, 2(4), 329–336.

6. Thompson, A., Meah, D., Ahmed, N., Conniff-Jenkins, R., Chileshe, E., Phillips, C. O., Row, P. E. (2013). Comparison of the antibacterial activity of essential oils and extracts of medicinal and culinary herbs to investigate potential new treatments for irritable bowel syndrome. *BMC Complementary and Alternative Medicine*, 13, 338. Doi: 10.1186/1472-6882-13-338.

Chapter 26 – The "Petite" Questions

1. Samaritan's Purse International Relief (2017). "A Miraculous Day". August 21, 2014. Retrieved from https://www.samaritanspurse.org/article/samaritans-purse-doctor-recovered-from-ebola/ (accessed on May 11th, 2017).

2. Kaye, R. (October 6, 2014). How the Ebola drug ZMapp is made. Khon2 News. http://khon2.com/2014/10/06/how-the-ebola-drug-zmapp-is-made/ (accessed on May 11th, 2017).

3. Encyclopedia Wikipedia. ZMapp. Retrieved from https://en.wikipedia.org/wiki/Zmapp (accessed on May 11th, 2017).

4. American Diabetes Association (2017). Does Cinnamon Help Lower Blood Glucose? Retrieved from http://www.diabetes.org/food-and-fitness/food/what-can-i-eat/making-healthy-food-choices/does-cinnamon-help-lower-blood-glucose.html?referrer=https://www.google.com/ (accessed on May 11th, 2017).

ACKNOWLEDGEMENTS

I'd like to express immense gratitude to my father in heaven for bringing these great concepts to light through me.

To my amazing husband and our precious children, I'm grateful for your continual love and support, also through the writing of this book.

To my dad, the late Dr. A. O. C. Nettey-Marbell (1936-2017) and my mom, Mrs. Beatrice Nettey-Marbell, I'm forever thankful for the many opportunities you gave me while growing up, that have stirred within me a lifelong love for health and wellness. And to my wonderful siblings, your families, and my friends, I appreciate each one of you!

Finally, to my clients, thank you for challenging me daily to impact more in the area of health and wellness. Continue to take charge, and live well!

www.ingramcontent.com/pod-product-compliance
Lightning Source LLC
Chambersburg PA
CBHW062046270326
41931CB00013B/2967